# CHILDREN AND AIDS

# Clinical Practice

Number 19

*Judith H. Gold, M.D., F.R.C.P.(C)*
*Series Editor*

# CHILDREN AND AIDS

*Edited by*

## Margaret L. Stuber, M.D.

Assistant Professor of Psychiatry
University of California, Los Angeles

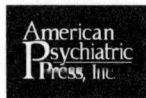

American
Psychiatric
Press, Inc.

Washington, DC
London, England

Note: The authors have worked to ensure that all information in this book concerning drug dosages, schedules, and routes of administration is accurate as of the time of publication and consistent with standards set by the U.S. Food and Drug Administration and the general medical community. As medical research and practice advance, however, therapeutic standards may change. For this reason and because human and mechanical errors sometimes occur, we recommend that readers follow the advice of a physician who is directly involved in their care or the care of a member of their family.

Copyright © 1992 American Psychiatric Press, Inc.
ALL RIGHTS RESERVED
Manufactured in the United States of America on acid-free paper
First Edition 95  94  93  92  4  3  2  1

American Psychiatric Press, Inc.
1400 K Street, N.W., Washington, DC  20005

**Library of Congress Cataloging-in-Publication Data**
Children and AIDS  / edited by Margaret L. Stuber. — 1st ed.
    p.  cm. — (Clinical practice ; no. 19)
   Includes bibliographical references.
   ISBN 0-88048-199-4 (alk. paper)
   1. AIDS (Disease) in children.   2. AIDS (Disease) in children—
social aspects.    I. Stuber, Margaret L., 1953-  .  II. Series.
   [DNLM:   1. Acquired Immunodeficiency Syndrome—in infancy
& childhood.   W1 CL767J no. 19 / WD 308 C536]
RJ387.A25C46   1991
618.95'9792—dc20
DLC
for Library of Congress               91-4581
                                         CIP

**British Library Cataloguing in Publication Data**
A CIP record is available from the British Library.

# Contents

# Contributors

**Lynn S. Baker, M.D.**
Assistant Clinical Professor of Psychiatry, University of
California, Los Angeles, School of Medicine

**Anita L. Belman, M.D.**
Associate Professor of Neurology, School of Medicine, State
University of New York at Stony Brook

**Mary G. Boland, R.N., M.S.N.**
Director, AIDS Program, Children's Hospital of New Jersey,
Newark; and Associate in Pediatrics, University of Medicine
and Dentistry of New Jersey, New Jersey Medical School,
Newark

**Pim Brouwers, Ph.D.**
Head, Neuropsychology Unit, and Visiting Scientist, Pediatric
Branch, National Cancer Institute, National Institutes of Health,
Bethesda, Maryland

**Gina Brown, M.D.**
Clinical Instructor of Obstetrics and Gynecology, Columbia
University, College of Physicians and Surgeons; and Attending
Physician in Obstetrics and Gynecology, Harlem Hospital and
Medical Center, New York, New York

**Toni Cabat, M.S.W.**
Assistant Director of Social Work, Memorial Sloan Kettering
Cancer Center, New York, New York

**Mark Chaffin, Ph.D.**
Assistant Professor of Pediatrics, University of Arkansas School
of Medicine, Little Rock

**Lynn Czarniecki, R.N., M.S.N.**
Clinical Specialist, AIDS Program, Children's Hospital of New
Jersey, Newark

**Dennis W. Dickson, M.D.**
Associate Professor of Pathology (Neuropathology), Albert
Einstein College of Medicine, Bronx, New York

**Harold Ginzburg, M.D., J.D., M.P.H.**
Senior Medical Consultant, Bureau of Health Care Delivery
and Assistance, Health Resources and Services Administration;
and Professor of Preventive Medicine and Biometrics and
Clinical Professor of Psychiatry, Uniformed Services University
of the Health Sciences School of Medicine, Bethesda, Maryland

**Heidi J. Haiken, A.C.S.W.**
Social Work Services Coordinator, AIDS Program, Children's
Hospital of New Jersey, Newark

**The Reverend Ross B. Hildebrand, S.T.B.**
St. Peter's Episcopal Church, Bronx, New York

**Rose Huntzinger, Ph.D.**
Assistant Professor of Psychiatry and Human Behavior, Brown
University; and Clinical Child Neuropsychologist, Bradley
Hospital, East Providence, Rhode Island

**Heather Huszti, Ph.D.**
Clinical Assistant Professor of Psychiatry and Behavioral
Sciences, University of Oklahoma Health Sciences Center,
Oklahoma City

**Cheryl Koopman, Ph.D.**
Assistant Professor of Clinical Psychology, Columbia
University, College of Physicians and Surgeons; and HIV Center
for Clinical and Behavioral Studies, New York State Psychiatric
Institute, New York, New York

**Penelope K.G. Krener, M.D.**
Associate Professor of Psychiatry and Pediatrics and Chief,
Division of Child, Adolescent, and Family Psychiatry,
University of California, Davis

**Mhairi MacDonald, M.B.Ch.B., F.R.C.P.(E), D.C.H.**
Vice Chair of Neonatology, Children's National Medical Center;
and Professor of Pediatrics, George Washington University,
Washington, DC

**Holly A. Magaña, Ph.D.**
Lecturer, Program in Social Ecology, University of California
at Irvine

**J. Raul Magaña, Ph.D.**
Vice President of Buena Care and Research Division, Alta Med
Health Services Corporation, Los Angeles; and formerly with
the Orange County Health Care Agency, Orange, California

**Janet Mitchell, M.D., M.P.H.**
Assistant Professor of Clinical Obstetrics and Gynecology,
Columbia University College of Physicians and Surgeons; and
Director of Perinatal Medicine, Department of Obstetrics and
Gynecology, Harlem Hospital and Medical Center, New York,
New York

**Roberta Olson, Ph.D.**
Associate Professor of Pediatrics, University of Oklahoma
Health Sciences Center, Oklahoma City

**Lucretia Robertson**
Parishioner and Volunteer, St. Luke's Episcopal Church,
Montclair, New Jersey

**Mary Jane Rotheram-Borus, Ph.D.**
Associate Professor of Clinical Psychology, Columbia
University College of Physicians and Surgeons; and HIV Center
for Clinical and Behavioral Studies, New York State Psychiatric
Institute, New York, New York

**Margaret L. Stuber, M.D.**
Assistant Professor of Psychiatry, University of California,
Los Angeles

**John M. Watkins, Ph.D.**
Assistant Professor of Pediatrics and Psychiatry, University
of California, Los Angeles

**Sterling B. Williams, M.D.**
Professor of Clinical Obstetrics and Gynecology, Columbia
University College of Physicians and Surgeons; and Director,
Department of Obstetrics and Gynecology, Harlem Hospital
and Medical Center, New York, New York

# Introduction
## to the Clinical Practice Series

$O$ver the years of its existence the series of monographs entitled *Clinical Insights* gradually became focused on providing current, factual, and theoretical material of interest to the clinician working outside of a hospital setting. To reflect this orientation, the name of the Series has been changed to *Clinical Practice*.

The Clinical Practice Series will provide readers with books that give the mental health clinician a practical clinical approach to a variety of psychiatric problems. These books will provide up-to-date literature reviews and emphasize the most recent treatment methods. Thus, the publications in the Series will interest clinicians working both in psychiatry and in the other mental health professions.

Each year a number of books will be published dealing with all aspects of clinical practice. In addition, from time to time when appropriate, the publications may be revised and updated. Thus, the Series will provide quick access to relevant and important areas of psychiatric practice. Some books in the Series will be authored by a person considered to be an expert in that particular area; others will be edited by such an expert who will also draw together other knowledgeable authors to produce a comprehensive overview of that topic.

Some of the books in the Clinical Practice Series will have their foundation in presentations at an annual meeting of the American Psychiatric Association. All will contain the most recently available information on the subjects discussed. Theoretical and scientific data will be applied to clinical situations, and case illustrations will be utilized in order to make the material even more relevant for the practitioner. Thus, the Clinical Practice Series should provide educational reading in a compact format especially written for the mental health clinician–psychiatrist.

Judith H. Gold, M.D., F.R.C.P.(C)
*Series Editor*
*Clinical Practice Series*

# Clinical Practice Series Titles

**Treating Chronically Mentally Ill Women (#1)**
Edited by Leona L. Bachrach, Ph.D., and Carol C. Nadelson, M.D.

**Divorce as a Developmental Process (#2)**
Edited by Judith H. Gold, M.D., F.R.C.P.(C)

**Family Violence: Emerging Issues of a National Crisis (#3)**
Edited by Leah J. Dickstein, M.D., and Carol C. Nadelson, M.D.

**Anxiety and Depressive Disorders in the Medical Patient (#4)**
By Leonard R. Derogatis, Ph.D., and Thomas N. Wise, M.D.

**Anxiety: New Findings for the Clinician (#5)**
Edited by Peter Roy-Byrne, M.D.

**The Neuroleptic Malignant Syndrome and Related Conditions (#6)**
By Arthur Lazarus, M.D., Stephan C. Mann, M.D., and Stanley N. Caroff, M.D.

**Juvenile Homicide (#7)**
Edited by Elissa P. Benedek, M.D., and Dewey G. Cornell, Ph.D.

**Measuring Mental Illness: Psychometric Assessment for Clinicians (#8)**
Edited by Scott Wetzler, Ph.D.

**Family Involvement in Treatment of the Frail Elderly (#9)**
Edited by Marion Zucker Goldstein, M.D.

**Psychiatric Care of Migrants: A Clinical Guide (#10)**
By Joseph Westermeyer, M.D., M.P.H., Ph.D.

**Office Treatment of Schizophrenia (#11)**
Edited by Mary V. Seeman, M.D., F.R.C.P.(C), and Stanley E. Greben, M.D., F.R.C.P.(C)

**The Psychosocial Impact of Job Loss (#12)**
By Nick Kates, M.B.B.S., F.R.C.P.(C), Barrie S. Greiff, M.D., and Duane Q. Hagen, M.D.

**New Perspectives on Narcissism (#13)**
Edited by Eric M. Plakun, M.D.

**Clinical Management of Gender Identity Disorders in Children and Adults (#14)**
Edited by Ray Blanchard, Ph.D., and Betty W. Steiner, M.B., F.R.C.P.(C)

# Introduction

## Who Is Our Audience, and Why This Book

> In less than a decade, pediatric AIDS will become one of the leading causes of death in small children. In 1981, AIDS was a rare diagnosis in children, often confused with congenital immunodeficiency syndromes of childhood; by 1991, it has been estimated that worldwide most new cases of AIDS will occur in children. (Koop CE: Inaugural editorial. *Pediatric AIDS and HIV Infection: Fetus to Adolescent* 1:7, 1990)

*W*hen I was first asked to address the issue of children and AIDS for the American Psychiatric Press, I made an outline of the topics I felt were essential to a clinical understanding of this new and rapidly growing area. A colleague who saw the outline asked if I thought anyone would want to read a book that focused on so many discouraging topics: poverty, racism, drug abuse, prostitution, dying children, dementia. As the book has taken shape, I've reflected on that comment, determined to have the authors communicate the hope and progress that keeps them actively working in this field. I believe that energy comes through in their writing. My hope is that this book will be inspirational as well as educational for readers.

This book was written by and for individuals across the United States and from a multitude of disciplines. It encompasses the perspectives of law, social work, nursing, psychology, anthropology, neurology, obstetrics, neuropsychology, and neonatology, as well as psychiatry and child psychiatry. The common link for all these authors is an interest in the clinical issues raised by children and AIDS. Some chapters present research data, whereas others are primarily descriptive. Readers will find certain themes repeated from different perspectives. Together they present a gestalt of what clinicians who work with children and AIDS encounter.

I want to express my gratitude to the authors, who took time out from busy lives and careers to write the excellent and lucid chapters of this book. I also want to thank the reviewers, who carefully and critically assessed each chapter and worked with me in giving constructive suggestions to the authors. I hope they are pleased with the results of their efforts. Finally, I want to thank my husband, Larry Gail, and my administrative assistant, Margie Greenwald, for their understanding, support, and, above all, patience throughout the process of this book's conception, gestation, and delivery.

This book is dedicated to Aaron Barbakow and his parents, who have taught me so much about life and hope, as well as about pediatric AIDS.

Margaret L. Stuber, M.D.

# The Context of Pediatric HIV and AIDS

*Chapter 1*

# Vertical Transmission of HIV: Management of the Pregnant Mother and Her Infant

Mhairi MacDonald, M.B.Ch.B., F.R.C.P.(E), D.C.H.

*C*urrently in the United States, approximately 84% of new cases of acquired immunodeficiency syndrome (AIDS) in children result from vertical transmission from mother to infant (Centers for Disease Control 1991). Recent Centers for Disease Control data confirm the expected link between the size of the AIDS epidemic among women and the number of cases of pediatric AIDS (Centers for Disease Control 1991). Intrauterine infection with the human immunodeficiency virus (HIV) has been documented by analysis of fetal thymus, cord blood samples, and placental tissue (Lapointe et al. 1985). It has been suggested that intrapartum infection could occur during exposure to maternal blood and secretions at birth; however, most studies comparing natural birth versus cesarean section have not shown a difference in the transmission rate related to mode of delivery (Cowan et al. 1984; Minkoff et al. 1987). Transmission to the neonate via breast milk is also documented, although the practical importance of this route remains controversial (Oxtoby 1988).

Early studies, mostly retrospective or with a short postnatal follow-up period, indicated that between 40% and 60% of infants born to HIV-seropositive mothers became infected. Overall, subsequent prospective studies have yielded a more conservative estimate of between 25% and 40% (European Collaborative Study 1988; Hira et al. 1989; Italian Multicentre Study 1988). It has been suggested that the risk of a mother transmitting the virus to her fetus may be related to the severity of her own disease. A study of HIV-seropositive mothers in Kinshasa, Zaire, indicated that women with more advanced disease or with lower

3

T4 lymphocyte counts were more likely to transmit infection to their infants (Ryder et al. 1989). However, Goedert et al. (1989) did not find this correlation. Preliminary evidence also suggests that transplacental passage of maternal antibodies against select epitopes of HIV envelope protein gp-120 may play a protective role in preventing mother-to-infant transmission of HIV infection in full-term babies (Goedert et al. 1989; Rossi et al. 1989).

Although intravenous-drug use remains the primary route of maternal infection (42% of cases reported from July 1988 to June 1989), infection through heterosexual contact has been growing at a more rapid rate. From July 1988 to June 1989, 28% of children newly diagnosed with perinatally acquired AIDS were born to heterosexually infected mothers. Two-thirds of these mothers were known to have had sexual intercourse with a partner who used illicit intravenous drugs (Centers for Disease Control 1991).

Seroprevalence surveys reveal a dramatic disparity between urban and suburban or rural residents. Seroprevalence for HIV among infants born in inner New York City was almost eight times higher than seroprevalence among infants born in upstate New York (Novick et al. 1989). In Massachusetts, mothers giving birth in inner-city hospitals were almost 7 times more likely to bear seropositive children than their suburban or rural counterparts, and over 26 times more likely than suburban mothers alone (Hoff et al. 1988).

In this chapter, I describe a basic care plan for the confirmed or suspected HIV-infected pregnant woman and her newborn and discuss the pitfalls in the diagnosis of HIV infection in the young infant. I also briefly describe the natural history of vertically acquired HIV infection and some of the new drug research protocols that are now enrolling pregnant patients and small children.

## Identification and Management of Pregnant Women at Risk for HIV Infection

Routine patient histories taken at clinical facilities serving women at risk for HIV infection (including those who use intravenous drugs, have multiple sexual partners, and/or have sexual intercourse with intravenous-drug users) should include confidential questions designed to elucidate individual risk. Written and/or audiovisual materials should be available at these sites for patient self-education, in addition to culturally sensitive counseling on an individual basis.

Screening for HIV is strongly encouraged for women considered to be at risk. Those presenting for prenatal care are tested at initial presentation and retested in the late third trimester to rule out recent infection. Because many women do not know whether they have been exposed to HIV, universal screening should be considered in inner-city hospitals in areas with a high prevalence of positive serology. Several studies have found that when screening for HIV is limited to patients who self-report an at-risk status, up to 70% of HIV-positive mothers may not be identified (Krasinski et al. 1988; Landesman et al. 1987; Lindsay et al. 1989).

Experience to date indicates that, when approached in a sensitive manner with appropriate explanation of the need for the screen, the majority of pregnant women will readily agree to be tested. Confidentiality must be assured, and screening should be undertaken to ensure optimal care for the mother and her baby and not as an alternative to the use of universal precautions by the hospital staff.[1]

Patients who are identified as being HIV antibody positive on repeated enzyme-linked immunosorbent assay (ELISA) and confirmed by Western blot[2] should be counseled about their clinical status and its potential impact on their fetus. Counseling should address not only adaptation to HIV infection but also the psychodynamics of pregnancy, the anticipation of illness in the infant, and the management of drug addiction and chaotic life-style (James 1988). Referral for psychiatric consultation may be indicated. Referral of sexual partners for counseling and testing should be strongly encouraged, and the patient (and partner if possible) should be instructed how to correctly use a condom to avoid transmitting HIV to sexual partners who are not already infected. Those who are users of illicit intravenous drugs are encouraged to enter treatment programs and to avoid sharing needles and syringes.

---

[1]*Universal precautions* refer to the observance of isolation or infection control procedures at all times, rather than specifically with individuals suspected of HIV infection. Guidelines are specified for various hospital functions, including labor and delivery and inpatient psychiatric facilities. (See guidelines issued by the American Psychiatric Association and American Academy of Child and Adolescent Psychiatry.)

[2]ELISA is the term used for the enzyme immunoassay (EIA) serologic testing for antibody to HIV-1 virus. Serum samples that are repeatedly reactive to EIA for HIV-1 antibody are then retested with Western blot, a more specific serologic test for antibody to HIV-1, using protein electrophoresis.

## The Question of Abortion

Women who are identified as being HIV positive during the first or early second trimester of pregnancy are given the option of terminating the pregnancy. Minkoff and Schwarz (1986) stated that a patient whose fetus may develop AIDS should be entitled to the same option to terminate the pregnancy as the patient with a fetus with any other lethal disease. Currently, there is little available information regarding the percentage of HIV-positive pregnant patients who will elect to have an abortion. Lindsay et al. (1989) found that one of six of their patients who were identified as being HIV positive before the 24th week of pregnancy underwent a voluntary abortion. However, 40% of their HIV-positive patients did not present for prenatal care until after the 24th week of gestation. Selwyn et al. (1986) found no difference in the frequency of voluntary abortions related to the patient's HIV status among a group of women followed prospectively at a methadone clinic. Data from this study, and others quoted, indicate that there is a significantly higher incidence of elective abortion among HIV-positive women when they receive counseling before becoming pregnant.

In a more recent study, Selwyn et al. (1989) found that decisions to terminate pregnancies by HIV-positive women were based more on variables related to pregnancy (such as prior elective abortion and whether pregnancy had been planned) than on concerns about perinatal transmission of HIV. The authors emphasized that counseling of women infected with HIV must incorporate consideration of the sociocultural and behavioral context in which decision making about pregnancy takes place.

There is ongoing debate about whether pregnancy accelerates the progression of asymptomatic HIV infection in the mother to AIDS-related complex (ARC) or AIDS. More research is required to answer this question, particularly when the mother becomes pregnant at a relatively advanced stage of the disease. A study by Biggar et al. (1989) showed that CD4[3] cells in HIV-positive women appeared to be lost faster during pregnancy than in the postpartum period. However, HIV-infected nonpregnant controls were not included, thus only allowing the conclusion that CD4 counts of HIV-infected pregnant women tend to decrease

---

[3]CD4 is the receptor site associated with HIV infection. Human leukocytes with CD4 receptors are commonly called CD4 cells or T4 cells.

significantly more than in noninfected pregnant women during gestation, and that the decrease appears to be permanent in the infected women.

## Management of HIV-Infected Pregnant Women

Management of pregnant patients with HIV infection should include careful testing for other sexually transmitted diseases. All prenatal patients are tested for gonorrhea, syphilis, and hepatitis B at the first prenatal visit. Patients who are HIV positive show increased frequency and severity of these infections and other sexually transmitted diseases.

Many early symptoms that may indicate progression from asymptomatic HIV infection to ARC or AIDS, such as fatigue, shortness of breath, and anemia, are common in pregnancy. Thus, obstetricians must be alert to these nonspecific symptoms and signs. If the pregnant woman has either ARC or AIDS or develops these conditions during pregnancy, patient care is coordinated with an infectious disease specialist, immunologist, or internist. The usual treatments for many of the common opportunistic infections that develop in immunosuppressed patients have theoretical teratogenic risks. However, it is generally felt that the benefits of these drugs during pregnancy outweigh the risks (Minkoff 1987).

To date, there are no standard recommendations for the use or safety of zidovudine (AZT) in pregnancy. Although AZT is known to cross the placenta and to reach therapeutic blood levels in the fetus (Gillet et al. 1989), animal studies and in vitro testing have not shown changes that would indicate teratogenic effects.

There is no clear evidence of an increased risk of obstetric complications in HIV-positive patients, if the infection is their only risk factor. However, Koonin et al. (1989) studied pregnancy-associated maternal deaths due to AIDS in the United States. He reviewed 20 patients who died from AIDS during pregnancy or within a year of delivery and found that outcome for the infant was poor. Gloeb et al. (1988) found that only 15 of 50 HIV-positive patients had uncomplicated pregnancies. Neither of the above studies was controlled for the effects of factors such as use of illicit drugs and/or alcohol. The prospective study done by Selwyn et al. (1986), on the other hand, involved clients at a methadone clinic and found no increased risk of prematurity, stillbirth, or low-birth-weight infants in HIV-positive pregnant clients. Ninety percent of asymptomatic HIV-positive patients who delivered at a hospital in inner-city Atlanta had term live births (Lindsay et al. 1989). In a recent study, Minkoff et al.

(1990) found that HIV-positive women with low CD4 counts are at markedly increased risk of serious infections during pregnancy.

## General Care of Newborns at Risk for HIV Infection

HIV may be present in the blood, vaginal secretions, and amniotic fluid of asymptomatic infected women. Gloves should be worn when handling the newborn infant, until the infant is bathed with soap and water to remove blood and vernix. Universal precautions should then be conducted in a rational and sensitive manner (Centers for Disease Control 1987). In particular, mothers should understand that the use of these precautions does not label their baby as being infected with HIV.

When there is passage of thick meconium by the fetus, effective and safe aspiration of the airway is essential. For the past decade in the United States, the standard method of suctioning meconium from the mouth and trachea of the newborn has required the use of oral suction applied to a DeLee apparatus or directly to an endotracheal tube. The recognition of the possibility that HIV might be transmitted during oral suctioning for meconium has led to the use of carefully controlled mechanical suction for this purpose.

Mothers known or suspected to be infected with HIV should be permitted full access to their infants. Although there is good evidence that HIV can be transmitted via breast milk, this is probably an infrequent occurrence (Oxtoby 1988). Newly infected mothers or those with a severely compromised immune system may have higher titers of circulating virus and may, thus, be more likely to transmit virus in their milk. Currently, breast-feeding by HIV-positive women is not encouraged in the United States. However, the World Health Organization has recommended that women in developing countries continue to breast-feed because the potential benefits of breast-feeding, in an environment where poverty and unsanitary conditions prevail, may outweigh the risk of HIV infection by this route (World Health Organization 1985).

## Natural History of Vertically Acquired HIV

In infants vertically infected with HIV, early symptoms such as lymphadenopathy, hepatosplenomegaly, and persistent oral thrush do not usually appear until age 4–5 months (Nicholas et al. 1989). A cohort of 172 children born between 1979 and 1987 with perinatally acquired infection have been described by Scott et al. (1989). The children presented with symptomatic disease at a median age of 8 months (only 21% presented after age 2 years). The most common initial manifestations of disease were lymphoid interstitial pneumonia (17%), encephalopathy (12%), recurrent bacterial infections (10%), and Candida esophagitis (8%), for which the median survival periods from diagnosis were 72, 11, 50, and 12 months, respectively. Nine percent of the children had Pneumocystis carinii pneumonia at median age 5 months and had a median survival of only 1 month.

In this cohort, the median survival for all 172 children was 38 months from the time of diagnosis. Mortality was highest in the first year of life (17%). Early age at diagnosis and the first identifiable pattern of clinical disease were found to be independently related to duration of survival (Table 1–1). Scott et al. (1989) concluded that children with perinatally acquired HIV infection have a very poor prognosis, and that most become symptomatic before age 1 year. They emphasize the importance of early diagnosis, because there is only a short interval in which to initiate prophylactic or antiviral treatment before progressive disease begins.

## Diagnosis of HIV Infection in Neonates and Young Infants

The HIV antibody status of all newborns at risk for infection (in areas of high prevalence, this may mean all newborns) should be assessed as early in life as possible. There are no disease-specific clinical markers for HIV infection in the newborn period. In many cases, the mother is not aware that she is infected, frequently because she has received little or no prenatal care. The infant then becomes the index case for a potentially sick and dying family unit.

Transplacental transfer of maternal HIV antibodies renders early postnatal diagnosis of HIV infection in the newborn problematic. However, early identification of the infected infant is vital both to produce accurate disease surveillance data and to ensure that appropriate treatments and services are provided for the infant and family at the earliest possible juncture. Our current inability to identify the infected infant

**Table 1–1.** Incidence of HIV-1 infection, age at diagnosis, and survival in a cohort of children, according to pattern of HIV-1–associated disease

| Disease pattern | Patients with pattern | | Age (months) at diagnosis of pattern | | Median survival as first pattern (months) |
| | at any time (months) (%) | as first pattern | at any time (median) (range) | as first pattern | |
|---|---|---|---|---|---|
| Pneumocystis carinii pneumonia | 22 (14) | 14 (9) | 5 (3–61) | 5 (3–61) | 1 |
| Lymphoid interstitial pneumonia | 48 (30) | 27 (17) | 13 (5–81) | 14 (5–60) | 72 |
| Recurrent bacterial infections | 29 (18) | 16 (10) | 10 (1–39) | 9 (1–39) | 50 |
| Candida esophagitis | 24 (15) | 13 (8) | 19 (3–84) | 18 (3–84) | 12 |
| Cardiomyopathy | 23 (14) | 0 (0) | 22 (6–84) | | |
| Encephalopathy | 26 (16) | 20 (12) | 9 (1–89) | 9 (1–24) | 11 |
| Nephropathy | 14 (9) | 4 (2) | 39 (13–90) | 48 (13–78) | 5 |

*Note.* One hundred four children had at least one of the seven HIV-1–associated patterns of disease. Ten of these children were excluded from this table because it was not possible to ascertain which disease pattern had occurred first.
*Source.* Reproduced with permission from Scott GB, Hutto C, Makuch RW, et al: Survival in children with perinatally acquired human immunodeficiency virus type 1 infection. N Engl J Med 321:1791–1796, 1989.

leads to false "labeling" of noninfected babies and can result in serious social and developmental sequelae for the infant and misuse of scarce and expensive health care resources. Ethical issues arise when there is potential benefit to a truly infected infant from involvement in a treatment study with significant toxic side effects. It is difficult to justify the enrollment of an uninfected infant, with positive HIV serology on the basis of passively acquired maternal antibodies, in a potentially toxic Phase 1 or 2 drug treatment research project because there is no way of differentiating the infant from a truly infected infant.

The early identification of children with vertically acquired HIV is becoming increasingly more vital as standardized treatment regimens are introduced for the complications of HIV infection in young children and hospital and community services are developed that improve the quality of life for the infected child. This has led many health care professionals who care for newborns to feel that screening all newborns in inner-city hospitals for HIV should be routine. Knowing the infant's serologic status, despite its diagnostic limitations, allows for the organization and monitoring of optimal follow-up care. This is particularly important because the mother's life-style frequently places attendance for follow-up very low in her priorities.

Immunological abnormalities are not a sufficiently sensitive or specific marker on which to base a diagnosis of vertically acquired HIV infection. The principal laboratory abnormalities associated with HIV infection in adults—the reversal of the CD4-to-CD8 ratio and the decrease in the absolute number of CD4 cells—also occur in children. However, their appearance is frequently delayed. Young infants, in particular, may develop opportunistic infections indicative of AIDS in the presence of normal CD4 counts, and the organisms involved are often those that occur with significant frequency in sick non-HIV-infected premature infants, for example, *Candida* species and cytomegalovirus. Because those at highest risk for HIV infection in pregnancy are also highly at risk for premature delivery and are frequently abusing alcohol and other substances that can produce immune suppression in the infant, the pattern of opportunistic infection is not usually helpful in detecting the HIV-infected premature infant.

Serum immune globulins are frequently elevated in HIV-infected infants and children, and the increase is sometimes detected as early as age 4–6 months (Falloon et al. 1989; McNamara 1989). Delayed skin hypersensitivity is difficult to interpret in young infants, and responses to immunization and mitogen- or antigen-induced lymphocyte proliferation in vitro are usually not abnormal early in the course of infection or in the asymptomatic infant.

Maternal immunoglobulin G (IgG) antibody persists in infants for a median of over 10 months postnatally, and in some cases lingers for up to 18 months postnatally (European Collaborative Study 1988). If a mother develops infection close to the end of pregnancy and the fetus is delivered within the "window" period before maternal antibody response commences, a false-negative screen for HIV may result in the young infant. Paradoxically, this infant may be at increased risk of acquiring vertical HIV infection because of the presumed early viremia in the mother and lack of maternal immune response. It is likely that very premature infants (24–30 weeks gestational age) are not in utero long enough to receive a significant aliquot of transplacental antibodies.

At this time, no single test can identify all infants with HIV infection, and many of the available tests are expensive, require considerable expertise, are time consuming, and are only available in research laboratories. Several are outlined below.

1. Recovery of an infectious agent in culture has traditionally been the "gold standard" for proving an etiologic relationship. The requirement for a large quantity of blood (20–30 ml) initially made the technique unsuitable for small infants. However, recent improvements in the methodology permit successful recovery of HIV from as little as 2 ml of blood. Unfortunately, the overall sensitivity of the test is difficult to assess, and it may only detect up to 50% of infected infants (Cowan et al. 1988; Ulrich et al. 1988).

2. Detection of virus-specific DNA or RNA, using the nucleic acid hybridization technique, is a rapid, sensitive, and specific approach to the detection of viruses, particularly those that initiate a latent infection or are difficult to grow on tissue culture. Traditional methods of nucleic acid hybridization are not sufficiently sensitive to detect HIV-specific DNA in peripheral blood cells. However, polymerase chain reaction (PCR) amplifies the HIV-specific DNA so that its detection by hybridization becomes possible (Ou et al. 1988). Initial reports suggest that PCR shows great promise for the early diagnosis of vertically acquired HIV infection (Laure et al. 1988; Rogers et al. 1989).

3. The technique of in vitro antibody production is based on the assumption that if the infant is truly infected with HIV (and beyond the

"window" period), he or she will have initiated antibody production. Thus, when the infant's peripheral blood mononuclear cells are cultured in the presence of mitogens, HIV antibodies are detected in the tissue culture supernatant. Amadori et al. (1988) reported that cultured lymphocytes from 14 of 16 infected infants produced HIV antibodies detectable by Western blot.

4. Preliminary data suggest that measurement of the nonspecific markers $\beta_2$-microglobulin and neopterin can be helpful in identifying infants with HIV infection, particularly when the determinations are repeated over time (Chan et al. 1990).

It has recently been reported that the presence of antibodies to certain epitopes of gp-120 in pregnant women with HIV infection appears to confer protection to the fetus against transplacental infection with HIV (Goedert et al. 1989; Rossi et al. 1989). In the future, these antibody studies may provide a means to assess the risk of transmission of HIV from an individual mother to her fetus and perhaps facilitate decisions regarding the institution of prophylactic antiviral treatment in the mother or infant.

## Status of Antiviral Therapy in the Prevention and Treatment of Vertically Acquired HIV Infection

Until recently, the management of HIV-infected children was limited to supportive care (e.g., nutrition, passive immunization, and antibiotics). It has now been demonstrated that continuous intravenous administration of AZT can produce consistent and dramatic symptomatic improvement in pediatric patients presenting with neurodevelopmental abnormalities. In the patients reported by Pizzo et al. (1988), improvements other than those in central nervous system function were also noted during treatment with AZT by continuous infusion. These improvements included subjective changes (e.g., improved appetite, weight gain, and increased activity) and objective changes (e.g., decreased lymphadenopathy and/or hepatosplenomegaly, decreases in immunoglobulin levels, and increases in CD4 cell number). In a significant number of children treated with AZT, the degree of neurodevelopmental improvement appeared to be independent of whether other beneficial changes occurred in the patient's immune status or risk of opportunistic infection.

Intermittent oral therapy has been shown to produce beneficial effects in children with advanced HIV disease (McKinney et al. 1991), despite the short half-life of AZT (1–1.5 hours in infants older than age 30 days, but younger than age 3 months; 2–2.5 hours in infants younger than age 30 days [Boucher et al. 1989]). This means that with intermittent administration, a significant portion of time may be spent with blood levels less than the minimum necessary to inhibit HIV replication (1 µM/L). In this study (McKinney et al. 1991), 88 children were given a 180 mg/m$^2$ dose of AZT orally every 6 hours. Marked improvement was observed in weight gain, cognitive function (primarily in children younger than age 3 years), serum and cerebrospinal fluid (CSF) P-24 antigen, and the proportion of CSF cultures that were negative for HIV. As in adults, lower dosages may be equally effective and have fewer side effects. A study (NIAID ACTG 128) is under way to compare AZT in doses of 180 mg/m$^2$ versus 90 mg/m$^2$ given four times per day (Fischl et al. 1990; Volberding et al. 1990).

The requirement for placement of a central venous line to administer continuous AZT adds the risks associated with these lines (in particular, infection) to the other known toxic effects of AZT, which include macrocytosis, anemia (necessitating replacement transfusions), and neutropenia. Toxic effects are related to dose and duration of therapy and are increased in patients with depressed helper T lymphocyte counts, hemoglobin values, or neutrophil counts at the start of therapy.

Even though AZT has beneficial effects while therapy is ongoing, deterioration of neurodevelopmental status occurs when treatment with the drug is discontinued. Current data in adults suggest that the prolonged use of AZT as the sole antiviral agent is limited by its toxic effect on bone marrow and possibly also by the development of viral resistance to the drug (Larder et al. 1989). Thus, the identification of agents that might be employed concurrently with AZT, to enhance and prolong the duration of beneficial effect and to limit or attenuate its toxicity, is of high priority. The Pediatric Branch of the National Cancer Institute and the National Institutes of Health–sponsored AIDS Clinical Trials Group are currently conducting and sponsoring studies in children to evaluate new antiretroviral agents, both when used alone and as part of combined therapeutic regimens. The drugs being studied include other dideoxynucleosides, such as 2'3'-dideoxycytidine (ddc) and dideoxyinosine (ddi), alone and in combination with AZT, and soluble CD4 (a molecularly cloned protein that binds to HIV and inhibits its ability to infect target cells). It is hoped that by emulating the successful experience with the development of current therapeutic strategies for childhood leukemia—by using several drugs in combination that inhibit HIV at different stages in its cycle of replication—effective treatment strategies with acceptable levels of toxic side effects will be developed.

Some of these agents may eventually prove effective in blocking the transmission of HIV from mother to child, when administered to the pregnant woman. Studies are already under way using AZT during the third trimester of pregnancy. The success of such "prophylactic" therapy, however, will depend on the currently unknown period during gestation when transplacental transmission most commonly occurs. The potential toxic side effects of a drug regimen will prove more problematic the earlier in gestation that therapy must commence.

## Priorities for the Future

In the coming decade, a nondefeatest attitude must be adopted to the development of effective preventive strategies to stem the spread of HIV among female adolescents and other women of reproductive age. These strategies must be designed to overcome and prevail against the formidable obstacles to reaching the high-risk population in the drug-abusing "underclass."

More reliable, but not excessively time-consuming or costly, diagnostic methods must be developed to allow early definitive diagnosis of HIV infection in the newborn and, thus, early triage of mothers and their infants into appropriate treatment programs. Also required is further documentation of clinicopathological correlations—more pooled biopsy and autopsy information on which to base earlier recognition of the manifestations of the complications of HIV disease and timely initiation of therapeutic interventions.

As the epidemic of pediatric HIV infection progresses, and as treatment regimens produce a positive impact on survival, the costs of care will increase. Available data demonstrate, on a per capita basis, that the cost of hospital care for a child with HIV infection is significantly higher than the cost of such care for an adult (Parrott 1991). Increased development and better organization of outpatient hospital, home-care, and community services for infected families should help to keep these costs to a minimum.

Finally, development of optimal care systems for the HIV-infected pregnant woman and her family involves well-orchestrated teamwork among all services involved. Thus, the obstetrician, pediatrician, psychiatrist, drug-abuse treatment specialist, social worker, researcher, community services provider, and all other key individuals involved must communicate with and recognize the roles of each of the other team members in the provision of the best possible care to the family unit devastated by HIV infection. Lines of communication must be clear, but must appropriately protect patient confidentiality. Members of the care network should maintain and share an up-to-date knowledge base on HIV infection in women and children and on effective preventive or therapeutic innovations.

# References

Amadori A, Giaquinto C, Zacchello F, et al: In-vitro production of HIV specific antibody in children at risk of AIDS. Lancet 1:852–854, 1988

Biggar RJ, Pahwa S, Minkoff H, et al: Immunosuppression in pregnant women infected with human immunodeficiency virus. Am J Obstet Gynecol 161:1239–1244, 1989

Boucher FD, Prober CC, Arvin AM, et al: A phase one study of zidovudine (AZT) in infants less than three months old, at risk for HIV infection (abstract WBO 2). Paper presented at the 5th International Conference on AIDS, Montreal, Quebec, Canada, June 1989

Centers for Disease Control: Recommendations for prevention of HIV transmission in health care settings. MMWR 36:3–18, 1987

Centers for Disease Control: HIV/AIDS surveillance report. Washington, DC, U.S. Government Printing Office, February 1991, pp 1–18

Chan MM, Campos JM, Josephs S, et al: $\beta_2$-Microglobulin and neopterin: predictive markers for human immunodeficiency virus type 1 infection in children? J Clin Microbiol 28:2215–2219, 1990

Cowan MJ, Hellman D, Chudwin D, et al: Maternal transmission of acquired immunodeficiency syndrome. Pediatrics 73:382–386, 1984

Cowan MJ, Walker C, Culver K, et al: Maternally transmitted HIV infection in children. AIDS 2:437–441, 1988

European Collaborative Study: Mother-to-child transmission of HIV infection. Lancet 2:1039–1043, 1988

Falloon J, Eddy J, Wiener L, et al: Human immunodeficiency virus infection in children. J Pediatr 114:1–30, 1989

Fischl MA, Parker CB, Pettinelli C, et al: A randomized controlled trial of a reduced daily dose of zidovudine in patients with the acquired immunodeficiency syndrome. N Engl J Med 323:1009–1014, 1990

Gillet JY, Garraffo R, Abrar D, et al: Fetoplacental passage of zidovudine. Lancet 1:269–327, 1989

Gloeb DJ, O'Sullivan NJ, Efantis J: Human immunodeficiency virus infection in women, I: the effects of human immunodeficiency virus on pregnancy. Am J Obstet Gynecol 159:756–761, 1988

Goedert JJ, Drummond JE, Minkoff H, et al: Mother-to-infant transmission of human immunodeficiency virus type 1: association with prematurity or low anti-gp 120. Lancet 2:1351–1354, 1989

Hira SK, Kamanga J, Bhat GJ, et al: Perinatal transmission of HIV-1 in Zambia. Br Med J 299:1250–1252, 1989

Hoff R, Berardi V, Weiblen B, et al: Seroprevalence of human immunodeficiency virus among childbearing women. N Engl J Med 318:525–530, 1988

Italian Multicentre Study: Epidemiology, clinical features, and prognostic factors of pediatric HIV infection. Lancet 2:1043–1045, 1988

James ME: HIV seropositivity diagnosed during pregnancy: psychosocial characterization of patients and their adaptation. Gen Hosp Psychiatry 10:309–316, 1988

Koonin LM, Ellerbrock TV, Atrash HK, et al: Pregnancy-associated deaths due to AIDS in the United States. JAMA 261:1306–1309, 1989

Krasinski K, Borkowsky W, Bebenroth D, et al: Failure of voluntary testing for human immunodeficiency virus to identify infected parturient women in a high-risk population (letter). N Engl J Med 318:185, 1988

Landesman H, Minkoff H, Holman S, et al: Serosurvey of human immunodeficiency virus infection in parturients. JAMA 258:2701–2703, 1987

Lapointe N, Michaud J, Pekovic D, et al: Transplacental transmission of HTLV-III virus. N Engl J Med 312:1325–1326, 1985

Larder BA, Darby G, Richman DD: HIV with reduced sensitivity to zidovudine (AZT) isolated during prolonged therapy. Science 243:1731–1734, 1989

Laure F, Rouzioux C, Veber F, et al: Detection of HIV 1 DNA in infants and children by means of the polymerase chain reaction in infants born to seropositive mothers. Lancet 2:538–541, 1988

Lindsay MK, Peterson HB, Feng TI, et al: Routine antepartum human immunodeficiency virus infection screening in an inner-city population. Obstet Gynecol 74:289–294, 1989

McKinney RE Jr, Maha MA, Louhor EM, et al: A multicenter trial of oral zidovudine in children with advanced human immunodeficiency virus disease. N Engl J Med 324:1018–1025, 1991

McNamara JG: Immunologic abnormalities in infants infected with human immunodeficiency virus. Semin Perinatol 13:35–43, 1989

Minkoff HL: Care of pregnant women infected with human immunodeficiency virus. JAMA 258:2714–2717, 1987

Minkoff HL, Schwarz RH: AIDS: time for obstetricians to get involved. Obstet Gynecol 68:267–268, 1986

Minkoff HL, Nanda D, Menez R, et al: Pregnancies resulting in infants with acquired immunodeficiency syndrome or AIDS-related complex: follow-up of mothers, children, and subsequently born siblings (part 1). Obstet Gynecol 69:288–291, 1987

Minkoff HL, Willoughby A, Mendez H, et al: Serious infections during pregnancy among women with advanced human immunodeficiency virus infection. Am J Obstet Gynecol 162:30–34, 1990

Nicholas SW, Sondheimer DI, Willoughby AD, et al: Human immunodeficiency virus infection in childhood, adolescence, and pregnancy: a status report and national research agenda. Pediatrics 83:293–308, 1989

Novick LF, Berns D, Stricof R, et al: HIV seroprevalence in newborns in New York State. JAMA 261:1745–1750, 1989

Ou C-Y, Kwok S, Mitchell SW, et al: DNA amplification for direct detection of HIV-1 in peripheral blood mononuclear cells. Science 239:295–297, 1988

Oxtoby MJ: Human immunodeficiency virus and other viruses in human milk: placing the issues in broader perspectives. Pediatr Infect Dis J 7:1825–1835, 1988

Parrott RH: Childhood HIV infection: the spectrum of costs. Journal of Acquired Immunodeficiency Syndromes 4:122–129, 1991

Pizzo PA, Eddy J, Falloon J, et al: Effect of continuous infusion of zidovudine (AZT) in children with symptomatic HIV infection. N Engl J Med 319:889–896, 1988

Rogers MF, Ou C-Y, Rayfield M, et al: Use of the polymerase chain reaction for early detection of the proviral sequences of human immunodeficiency virus in infants born to seropositive mothers. N Engl J Med 320:1649–1654, 1989

Rossi P, Moschese V, Broliden PA, et al: Presence of maternal antibodies to human immunodeficiency virus 1 envelope glycoprotein gp 120 epitopes correlates with the uninfected status of children born to seropositive mothers. Proc Natl Acad Sci USA 86:8055–8058, 1989

Ryder R, Nsa W, Hassig S, et al: Perinatal transmission of the human immunodeficiency virus type 1 to infants of seropositive women in Zaire. N Engl J Med 320:1637–1642, 1989

Scott GB, Hutto C, Makuch RW, et al: Survival in children with perinatally acquired human immunodeficiency virus type 1 infection. N Engl J Med 321:1791–1796, 1989

Selwyn PA, Schoenbaum EE, Davenny K, et al: Prospective study of human immunodeficiency virus infection and pregnancy outcomes in intravenous drug users. JAMA 261:1289–1294, 1986

Selwyn PA, Carter RJ, Schoenbaum EE, et al: Knowledge of HIV antibody status and decisions to continue or terminate pregnancy among intravenous drug users. JAMA 261:3567–3571, 1989

Ulrich PP, Busch MP, El-Beik T, et al: Assessment of human immunodeficiency virus expression in cocultures of peripheral blood mononuclear cells from healthy seropositive subjects. J Med Virol 25:1–10, 1988

Volberding PA, Lagakos SW, Koch MA, et al: Zidovudine in asymptomatic human immunodeficiency infection. N Engl J Med 322:941–949, 1990

WHO recommendations for assisting in the prevention of perinatal transmission of human T-lymphocyte virus Type II/lymphadenopathy–associated virus and acquired immunodeficiency syndrome. MMWR 34:721–726, 731–732, 1985

Chapter 2

# The African American Community

Gina Brown, M.D.
Janet Mitchell, M.D., M.P.H.
Sterling B. Williams, M.D.

*E*pidemiologists, the federal government, and social and scientific researchers have been slow to address the effect of race and culture on the acquired immunodeficiency syndrome (AIDS) epidemic. Whether looking at survival rates, age at diagnosis, route of infection, or gender, African Americans have been disproportionately affected by this illness (Bakeman et al. 1986).

The epidemiology of infection with the human immunodeficiency virus (HIV) has been well described. Although African Americans compose only 12% of the population of the United States, they make up nearly 25% of reported AIDS cases (Centers for Disease Control 1989a). The current estimation is that the rate of HIV infection in African Americans is three times higher than that for whites. Unlike for males, as the absolute numbers of infected females and children increase, the overwhelming percentage are of either African American or Hispanic descent (Centers for Disease Control 1988, 1989a; Selik et al. 1988b). Most children infected during the perinatal period (80% of the total number of children with the disease) are from these ethnic groups, which include the nation's poorest citizens. Among heterosexual men, African Americans and Hispanics account for 70% of AIDS cases (Centers for Disease Control 1989a; Selik et al. 1988a, 1988b).

For the majority of men, women, and children from minority groups, HIV infection can be linked to drug use (Bakeman et al. 1986; Centers for Disease Control 1988, 1989a, 1989b; Selik et al. 1988a, 1988b). Minority status coupled with poverty in these individuals creates serious and complicated problems for their families, for the communities from which they come, and for the providers of their medical care. To compre-

hend the true impact of this disease on these families, one must understand the interrelationships of poverty, drug use, race, ethnicity, and
culture. AIDS has placed in sharp focus the need for more detailed data
about the effects of these variables on the lives and life-styles of these
families. In the absence of such data, the development of strategies to
provide care and to prevent the spread of the disease are difficult to
construct. To a large extent, the success, or lack of success, of current
strategies for treatment or prevention of HIV disease in the African
American community confirms this thesis.

## HIV and Access to Health Care

The picture of HIV in African Americans is a portrait of the urban poor.
The majority of African Americans who are infected with HIV reside in
the underprivileged areas of disintegrating urban centers. In addition to
poverty, drug use in these communities is rampant. The morbidity associated with drug use alone may complicate the illnesses associated with
HIV. The disorganization associated with the drug abuser's life-style
makes negotiating the system of health care and social services even
more difficult.

The poverty of families forces them to rely on the public sector of
the medical system for care. Nationally, public general hospitals or
public health clinics provide a disproportionate amount of care for all
HIV-infected patients and most of the medical care for minorities with
AIDS. Such institutions must rely on local tax levy funds to subsidize
medical care for those without health insurance. As a result, they are
chronically embattled, underfinanced, and understaffed. Unfortunately,
because the AIDS epidemic has occurred at a time of local as well as
national financial deficits, the entire system of public health and medical
care in those areas where HIV is most prevalent has been placed in great
jeopardy.

Medical care for the poor remains a major unsolved problem of the
nation's health care delivery system. As many as 40 million Americans
have no means to pay for medical care, and many more are seriously
underinsured. With its escalating cost, the ability to pay for that care has
become an increasing predictor of access to high-quality attention. HIV
infection presents a stark vision of the problems of the poor of this nation
who need medical care.

Medicaid, the principal source of health care financing for the poor, is organized as such a complicated bureaucracy that it can be negotiated successfully by only the most socially organized. HIV-infected African Americans, especially children, may lead lives disorganized by substance abuse and poverty. Therefore, the preventive health care that is important for everyone, particularly those who are infected with HIV, is underutilized by the African American population.

Health behaviors also differ for those with minority status (Levin 1984). For example, minorities commonly use medical care facilities only at times of perceived medical crisis. Belief in the value of health maintenance and preventive care develops only with rising educational and income status. Cultural beliefs may also have an impact on the adherence to defined medical regimens (Flaskerud and Rush 1989; Levin 1984; Marin 1989). The role of family, well-meaning grandparents, indigenous healers, and other community leaders may influence one's ability to follow the recommendations of health care providers. Religion plays a prominent role in most minority communities (Levin 1984). Faith in the "Almighty" often supersedes faith in man (medicine). These community resources can be a tremendous resource for strength and survival, but if not understood and appropriately utilized by the more traditional agencies, they can also be a source of enormous conflict.

Mistrust of government agencies, rooted in difficulties encountered for generations in their attempts to use them, also creates obstacles to the provision of appropriate medical services in the minority community. Involvement in illegal activities such as drug use will, of course, heighten this mistrust.

HIV infection is evolving into a chronic disease requiring complicated and disciplined therapy regimens. Compliance with treatment schedules requires considerable family organization and stability, often not found in families besieged by poverty, poor education, and inadequate housing. The energy required to survive may preclude the ability of persons to keep repeated clinic visits or to follow complicated drug schedules for themselves or their children.

Programs and agencies that have had success in reaching this population have learned to tap into this energy and survival instinct. Flexibility and understanding are necessary requirements to forge constructive liaisons with this population and to achieve the goal of improved access to health and social services.

# Perception of Risk

Recognizing the risk of HIV infection represents another barrier to the access to adequate care. There is a generalized perception in the African American community that AIDS is a disease of homosexual white males (Bouknight and Bouknight 1988; Flaskerud and Rush 1989; Mays and Cochran 1988; Peterson and Marin 1988). For the poverty-stricken African American community at risk, crime, drug use, and prostitution are day-to-day realities that are of immediate concern. The risk of HIV infection is just one problem among a multitude of others. The immediate issues of food, shelter, child care, and negotiating the system to obtain these things are of much greater importance.

Many HIV-infected women who are not themselves directly involved in drug use have innocently or consciously had sexual relationships with men who have been drug users and are HIV infected. In some low-income communities where the prevalence of HIV infection is high, simple residence in the community places sexually active women and men at risk for heterosexual transmission of the virus. Despite the fact that sexual transmission as a source of infection is growing rapidly, women may not see their partner's risky behavior as endangering their own lives (Marin 1989; Mays and Cochran 1988; Scott et al. 1985).

The reality of acquiring AIDS is often not considered until individuals actually become symptomatic. Women in particular may be more concerned with the maintenance of the family structure and may not become aware of their own infection status until they have a child who is infected and symptomatic (Scott et al. 1985). The ability to cope then becomes a function of the person's involvement with drugs and established relationships with family and friends. By not focusing solely on the disease of AIDS, these families may have a much more realistic outlook on the disease (Mays and Cochran 1987). Many middle-class infected individuals become "obsessed" with their infection. Poor urban communities must prioritize their life stresses. HIV becomes only one of many things that are of equal importance. Because this is a population that has traditionally been hard hit by whatever new health crisis may come along, African Americans see HIV as just one more burden to bear.

However, the perception of HIV as a "gay man's" disease allows African American men and women to avoid addressing their own risk as an issue (DiClemente et al. 1988; Mays and Cochran 1987). Occasional drug use with needle sharing is not seen as risky behavior. Lack of knowledge about a sexual partner's risk allows women to assume that they are not at risk (Mays and Cochran 1988). As a result, women may neglect their own health care and that of their children until symptoms emerge.

Homophobia presents a substantive barrier to risk perception in minority communities. Unlike for white men, for whom the predominant risk behavior for infection is homosexual or bisexual behavior, for minority men the percentage who admit homosexual or bisexual behavior approximately equals the percentage who admit drug use. The sexual activity that may occur during incarceration is dismissed on release into the community. Attitudes toward insertive versus receptive anal or oral sex create mental barriers to perceived risk of these behaviors. Public health messages that focus on vaginal-penile intercourse and receptive anal intercourse as risk factors allow women who may practice other behaviors to deny their own risks for HIV infection. Men who practice insertive anal sex may perceive no risk to themselves or their sexual partners. All of these factors help explain the recent increase in the rates of HIV infection among women and children (Williams 1986).

Within the past several years, an entirely new addiction has appeared in this country. Cocaine in its inexpensive form—crack, a far more destructive and terrifying drug—has swept urban low-income communities. Although heroin addiction was primarily found in men, cocaine and/or crack addiction is increasingly found in young women. Young female crack addicts are widely reported to use prostitution as a means of obtaining funds to support their habit. Many have sexual contact with men who are or who have been intravenous-drug users. Although precise estimates of the number of women infected by this route are not yet available, clearly this mechanism represents a new risk factor for HIV transmission.

## Education and Risk Reduction

Educational efforts regarding AIDS prevention have been largely delivered by the homosexual white community. The result is that the education is perceived as being relevant only to that group. This renders the health messages essentially ineffective in the African American community because the individuals who are delivering the information are not seen as credible (Williams 1986). A study that examined sexual attitudes and perceived risk of HIV infection (Mays and Cochran 1988) showed that 50% of the surveyed group of African American female college students felt that they had no risk of being exposed to the virus. Thirty percent had done nothing to change their behavior to prevent infection with HIV or any other sexually transmitted disease. The reception of efforts to educate the general public may be more closely related to the cultural relevance of the message than to the educational level or socioeconomic status of the recipient.

Differences between racial and ethnic groups and the many subcultures within these groups cannot be discounted. American-born African Americans have different beliefs from Caribbean-born African Americans. New York Puerto Ricans are a world apart from Los Angeles Mexicans. Native Americans and Pacific Islanders will not be reached by messages targeted to other ethnic groups (Williams 1986).

Any discussion of AIDS risk reduction must include an emphasis on condom use and contraception. These emotionally charged issues must be addressed in a culturally relevant fashion that respects beliefs commonly held among minorities. Childbearing is highly valued in minority communities (Gould 1984). Moreover, male domination is often absolute in areas of sexual behavior and contraceptive practices. The fear of "genocide," especially as it relates to family planning and use of contraception, still exists in African American communities. A study of fear of genocide among African Americans found that younger African Americans were more fearful of family-planning programs than older African Americans, and African American males were more suspicious than African American females. Even college-educated African Americans held these fears (Gould 1984).

The differences between male and female attitudes toward family planning in recent years have been dramatic. In 1984, Gould described the success of a group of minority women in reopening federally funded family-planning clinics that were forced to close by groups of "militant" African American men. Although published in 1984 with no reference to the AIDS crisis, Gould's suggestion to evaluate the appropriateness of certain messages about contraception is even more important today. For many women from minority communities, the suggestion to delay or terminate a pregnancy may be completely unacceptable to them or their partners. Messages about condom use targeted to women or men may conflict with their wishes to bear children or to father a child (Ralph 1986). Information targeted just to women is ineffective because, traditionally, men make the decision about condom use.

## Research Efforts

When the AIDS epidemic was recognized, research efforts were focused on the pharmacokinetics of treatment regimens that would slow progression of the disease or prevent the opportunistic infections associated with the immune-compromised state. Entry into the studies was limited, and as a result, very little information is available about the effects of many of these modalities on the drug-using population and on minorities and women in general. The ever-growing population of women who are HIV infected remains largely unstudied.

AIDS treatment study protocols are often located in centers away from those that traditionally serve the poor, undereducated, or drug-using populations. Access to the research programs requires that prospective participants are educated about their availability and savvy enough to understand how to negotiate the system in order to be enrolled.

Funds devoted to AIDS research are usually awarded to large educational institutions that have a history of obtaining monies from the federal government. These may not be institutions that provide care for large numbers of African Americans who are HIV infected. Because these individuals are often uninsured or underinsured, they do not have access to the same levels of care as their white counterparts. As a result, the information obtained from these efforts may not reflect the concerns and health responses of African Americans.

The gay male community continues to be the most organized lobbying effort for research devoted to AIDS treatment. As a result of lack of education, ethnic concerns remain largely unheard. Efforts targeted toward women seem to be focused around reproductive issues. This can be misconstrued as genocide by a community that has been traditionally mistrustful of government efforts to conduct research about them.

Another concern African Americans may have is the impact of data interpretation by researchers who may not understand the many cultural and racial issues that affect the information obtained in the studies (Banks et al. 1967). This may also affect accurate diagnoses of the mental illnesses that have been related to HIV infection. The formality many African Americans exhibit when presented with a white interviewer or health care provider may be misinterpreted as depression or, in severe cases, indicative of a thought disorder (Jones and Grey 1986). The fact that these misinterpretations can occur may make African Americans reluctant to participate in research efforts.

## Social Supports

Traditional social supports may not be available during times of stress and illness to African Americans who are HIV infected. Recognition of the illness means that individuals have admitted to socially unacceptable behaviors such as drug abuse, homosexuality, or promiscuity. Although African American churches may organize the community around illness or hardship among its members, it has provided very little open support for HIV-infected African Americans (Levin 1984). African Americans remain particularly intolerant of homosexuality. Some of those beliefs may be rooted in the church. Drug abuse and sexual promiscuity are also seen as "sinful" behavior. Situations such as illness, homelessness, and the need for social services that have traditionally resulted in a rallying effort by the African American church do not seem to be so inspiring when the person involved is HIV infected.

Many HIV-infected individuals who would previously have relied on their families or extended families for support are reluctant to "go home" when their hardship is related to AIDS. The profound guilt levied on them by themselves, their families, and their communities makes requesting help particularly difficult. The association of "sin" with their illness leads many to believe that they are "deserving" of their illness. As a result, many African Americans will only seek health care when their symptoms are far advanced.

Public and social services for AIDS victims include a "buddy" system, home care, and support groups. African Americans in need may not avail themselves of these services because they are often founded by organizations for homosexual individuals. Homosexual African American men may not have access to these services because they are frequently located outside the communities in which they live. The lack of culturally and ethnically focused public supports leaves many African Americans without such services. Ostracism by their own community results in the same.

## Counseling

Providing counseling and psychological support for African American patients remains a controversial issue in all illnesses. The stigmatization of AIDS, especially in the African American community, means that many individuals at risk will not come forward for counseling or testing.

As rumors of mandatory testing, partner notification, and placement of results in the medical record circulate, persons who may be symptomatic may not come forward for early treatment (Fordyce et al. 1989). They fear that the association of their route of infection with illegal or socially unacceptable activities may become known. The guilt associated with the behaviors that led to HIV infection results in a "this is my fault anyway" attitude and precludes the use of the available services. Many individuals feel that they are being justly punished for their behaviors.

Cultural differences in the perception of psychiatric illnesses have been well documented. Schizophrenia and psychosis tend to be over-diagnosed in African Americans, whereas the affective disorders are underrecognized (Jones and Grey 1986). Ethnic differences in the presentation of symptoms may also affect diagnoses. Remoteness and formality in dealing with white professionals may be misconstrued as an attempt to cover a thought disorder or psychotic process as opposed to the culturally traditional way of handling oneself among white strangers (Jones and Grey 1986). The unwillingness to share feelings with strangers may cause depressive disorders to be underdiagnosed because the patient may not be able to openly express feelings. The disorder may also be overdiagnosed in some instances when lack of communication is interpreted as flat affect or underlying hostility (Jones and Grey 1986).

Group counseling sessions may be especially unsuccessful when focused toward HIV infection in African Americans. Many continue to be linked to drug counseling at methadone maintenance centers. The instruments used for psychological assessment of addicts do not account for diversity in race, ethnicity, age, and drug use. The standardization of psychological assessment tools toward middle-class white norms leads to misinformation, misdiagnosis, and an incorrect assessment of the dynamics of the individuals within the group. The presumption that all individuals within the group are able to communicate their feelings in an open forum may be culturally invalid. Preconceived notions about drug use and minorities by the counselor may also adversely affect the usefulness of this forum in helping African Americans understand and cope with the impact of HIV infection on their lives.

The perceived ability of the counselor to understand the plight of the African American patient profoundly affects the success of psychotherapy (Banks et al. 1967). The inability of the therapist to understand may be presumed by the patient when the therapist is socially or racially different from the patient.

If group sessions are to be attempted, they must distinguish between women who became infected through their own drug use and women who became infected as a result of heterosexual transmission. African American women who are not drug users are often reluctant to identify themselves with women who are. Women who have used drugs often see HIV as part of the destiny of their lives. Infected individuals who do not use intravenous drugs express anger related to the "why me" concept, whereas those who use intravenous drugs often feel that they deserve their plight.

Groups must also distinguish between men who are infected through drug use and men who are infected because of sex with other men. This becomes complicated when one distinguishes men who have sex with other men while incarcerated from men who have sex with other men because of sexual preference or for the sake of survival (prostitution).

The educational counseling that accompanies HIV testing may also be affected by the patient's perception of whether the counselor can relate to his or her life-style (Mays and Cochran 1987; Williams 1986). In the case of African Americans and other minorities, white counselors may not be able to effectively deliver the educational message simply because the clients assume that they cannot. The health educator's use of "medicalese" and a lack of understanding of culturally and ethnically associated sexual behaviors can also inhibit the clients' incorporation of the information.

## Looking Toward the Future

The spectrum of HIV disease in the African American community is firmly rooted in all the risk behaviors, but drug abuse and heterosexual transmission account for percentages in excess of those of the white community. Any attempt to control this epidemic must begin with education and counseling programs that are culturally and ethnically sensitive, coupled with a service component to address the immediate needs of the person infected. Drug treatment programs must be expanded to include counseling for HIV prevention and primary health care. Programs must be expanded and their scope broadened to include treatment for crack abuse. Models for therapeutic intervention must be based on the realities of the communities from which the persons come. Family-planning programs and other programs that target women must be cautious in their approach and careful not to be perceived by the community as delivering coercive messages.

Better knowledge about the norms, attitudes, and behaviors of the African American populations most at risk is badly needed. To formulate and target appropriate interventions that will have an impact on the spread of the infection, an understanding of the differences and similarities among populations is essential. Inclusion of members from these populations in formulating strategies is not only critical but will expedite the process by which effective interventions can be implemented to halt the spread of HIV infection.

As HIV becomes a chronic disease with a longer survival period, the mental health field will play an increasingly important role. Providing appropriate support programs and interventions for the African American community will be essential to its emotional and mental stability. It is imperative that funds be appropriated and that attention be given to understanding this infection as it relates to the African American community. The continued increase in the rates of infection among minorities, especially drug users, women, and children, is the price paid for not understanding the impact of race, culture, and ethnicity on life-style, sex and drug-using behaviors, and community norms.

## References

Bakeman R, Lumb JR, Smith DW: AIDS statistics and the risk for minorities. AIDS Res 2:249–252, 1986

Banks G, Berenson B, Carkhuff R: The effects of counselor race and training upon the counseling process with Negro clients in initial interviews. J Clin Psychol 23:87–89, 1967

Bouknight RR, Bouknight LG: Acquired immunodeficiency syndrome in the black community: focusing on education and the black male. N Y State J Med 88:232–235, 1988

Centers for Disease Control: HIV-related beliefs, knowledge, and behaviors among high school students. MMWR 37:717–721, 1988

Centers for Disease Control: AIDS and human immunodeficiency virus infection in the United States: 1988 update. MMWR 38:1–38, 1989a

Centers for Disease Control: Update: acquired immunodeficiency syndrome—United States, 1981–1988. MMWR 38:229–237, 1989b

DiClemente RJ, Boyer CB, Morales ES: Minorities and AIDS: knowledge, attitudes, and misconceptions among black and Latino adolescents. Am J Public Health 78:55–57, 1988

Flaskerud JH, Rush CE: AIDS and traditional health beliefs and practices of black women. Nurs Res 38:211–215, 1989

Fordyce EJ, Sambula S, Stoneburner R: Mandatory reporting of human immunodeficiency virus testing would deter blacks and Hispanics from being tested (letter; comment). JAMA 262:349, 1989

Gould KH: Black women in double jeopardy: a perspective on birth control. Health Soc Work 9:96–105, 1984

Jones BE, Grey BA: Problems in diagnosing schizophrenia and affective disorders among blacks. Hosp Community Psychiatry 37:61–65, 1986

Levin JS: The role of the black church in community medicine. J Natl Med Assoc 6:477–483, 1984

Marin G: AIDS prevention among Hispanics: needs, risk behaviors, and cultural values. Public Health Rep 104:411–415, 1989

Mays VM, Cochran SD: Acquired immune deficiency syndrome and black Americans: special psychosocial issues. Public Health Rep 102:224–231, 1987

Mays VM, Cochran SD: Issues in the perception of AIDS risk and risk reduction activities by black and Hispanic/Latino women. Am Psychol 43:949–957, 1988

Peterson JL, Marin G: Issues on the prevention of AIDS among black and Hispanic men. Am Psychol 43:871–877, 1988

Ralph N, Spigner C: Contraceptive practices among female heroin addicts. Am J Public Health 76:1016–1017, 1986

Scott GB, Fischl MA, Klimas N, et al: Mothers of infants with the acquired immune deficiency syndrome. JAMA 253:363–366, 1985

Selik RM, Castro KG, Pappaioanou M: Distribution of AIDS cases by racial/ethnic group and exposure category, United States, June 1, 1981–July 4, 1988. MMWR 37:1–11, 1988a

Selik RM, Castro KG, Pappaioanou M: Racial/ethnic differences in the risk of AIDS in the United States. Am J Public Health 78:1539–1545, 1988b

Williams LS: AIDS risk reduction: a community health education intervention for minority high risk group members. Health Educ Q 13:407–421, 1986

*Chapter 3*

# Mexican-Latino Children

J. Raul Magaña, Ph.D.
Holly A. Magaña, Ph.D.

*T*he human immunodeficiency virus (HIV) has spread with alarming speed throughout Latino communities, and Latino children have succumbed to the disease at a disproportionately high and disturbing rate. Latino adults are three times more likely than the white population to contract the disease, and Latino children are seven times more likely to contract HIV than white children (Centers for Disease Control 1991). To understand why the disease has such a disproportionate impact on the Latino population, and Latino children in particular, it is necessary to understand the social and cultural factors that influence the spread of the disease and that make it such a challenging task to deliver effective education and preventive services to this population (Bennet 1987; Coates et al. 1984; Kinnier 1986; Martin and Vance 1984; Nelkin 1987).

In this chapter, we discuss the economic, cultural, and social factors that have influenced the spread of HIV in the Latino population in general and in Latino children in particular. We focus primarily on cultural factors relevant to Latinos of Mexican origin. Although many of the issues are similar for Latinos of different national origins (Hayes-Bautista and Chapa 1987; Klor de Alva 1988), our primary knowledge and experience is of Latinos of Mexican origin. We will also discuss the

This work was supported in part by the state of California, Office of AIDS, through the AIDS Community Education Project at the Health Care Agency, county of Orange, California. This chapter does not reflect the official position or policies of the county of Orange, the California Office of AIDS, or the University of California at Irvine. The authors bear sole responsibility for the contents of the article. The authors wish to thank Marta Borbon Ehling, Milagros Davila, Eunice Diaz, Jorge Camarillo, and Margaret L. Stuber, M.D., for helpful comments on an earlier draft of the chapter.

implications of social and cultural factors for designing effective education and prevention strategies to reduce the incidence of acquired immunodeficiency syndrome (AIDS) in Latino children.

## Social and Cultural Factors That Affect the Incidence of HIV Infection in Latino Children

### Economics and Demographics

The high fertility rates in the Latino community have important implications for the recent increases in pediatric AIDS cases among Latinos. Approximately 31% of Latinos are under age 15 years, compared to 21% of the remaining United States population. There are 111 live births for every 1,000 people in the Latino population, compared to 62 live births per 1,000 people in the non-Latino population (McCarthy and Burciaga 1988). High fertility rates coupled with other factors that contribute to a high rate of HIV infection in the Latino population have influenced the disproportionately high rates of pediatric AIDS.

The rapid spread of HIV in the Latino population is, in part, also affected by the large proportion of this population that is undocumented. It has been estimated that a sizable proportion of the Latino population in the United States may be undocumented (McCarthy and Burciaga 1988). The undocumented resident does not have health insurance, making access to medical care costly and difficult to locate and to obtain. Even when low-cost or free medical services are available in a particular area, undocumented residents may be reluctant to use the services for fear that their undocumented status will be discovered and that they will be deported (Hanh and Castro 1988). Therefore, AIDS education, treatment, and prevention programs for the Latino population must include an active outreach component so that the large segment of the population not currently being serviced by health care providers will be reached.

Poverty has an impact on all aspects of the health of the Latino population (Nyamathi and Vasquez 1989). The 1980 census indicates that almost 25% of Latino households are below the poverty level, compared to less than 10% of non-Latino, white households. This is probably a gross underestimate of the number of Latinos living in poverty because it does not take into account the many undocumented Latinos, the vast majority of whom are living on very limited incomes.

The low economic status of Latino families is associated with high rates of intravenous-drug use, which is implicated in 80% of Latino pediatric AIDS cases (Centers for Disease Control 1991). The low economic status of Latino families also carries with it limited access to health care services. Many of the jobs held by Latino laborers are not stable types of employment; therefore, laborers must make frequent moves to find employment. Moving frequently makes continuity of health care problematic (Chavez 1988). Furthermore, the family networks and support systems that usually play an important part in health care decisions are often broken up by frequent moves, contributing even more to the lack of adequate health care.

## Language and Education

The language skills and educational attainment of Latinos have a bearing on the health care and health education needs of the Latino community. The educational attainment of Latinos is markedly lower than that of the general population. It is estimated that the majority of Latino adults have fewer than 8 years of formal education, whereas this is true for only 10% of the general population. A sizable portion of recent Latino immigrants have fewer than 5 years of formal education (McCarthy and Burciaga 1988; Strategy Research Corporation 1989).

In addition to low levels of educational attainment, a large proportion of Latinos in the United States have limited mastery of the English language. The 1980 census indicates that approximately one-fifth of the Latino population speaks little or no English. This figure does not take into account the sizable population of undocumented Latino immigrants—the group that is most likely to have limited mastery of the English language. In fact, more recent data, based on samples that include Latinos with legal documentation as well as undocumented Latinos, estimate that between 63% and 78% of the Hispanic population in the United States speaks primarily Spanish at home and on social occasions (Strategy Research Corporation 1989).

The low levels of educational attainment in the Latino community coupled with limited mastery of the English language indicate that health education programs aimed at the general population will not be effective for a majority of the Latino population (Cole and Scribner 1974; Hochhauser 1987). This explains why early efforts to educate the general public regarding the prevention of the spread of AIDS may have had little effect on the Latino population and thus may be one factor contributing to the disproportionate number of AIDS cases among Latinos.

## Sexual Behavior and Attitudes

A number of beliefs and behaviors regarding sexuality result in patterns of sexual behavior that place the Latino population at a particularly high risk for the transmission of HIV and that specifically affect the spread of the virus to Latino women and children. These beliefs and behaviors have been documented most widely in the Mexican culture and may take on different characteristics in other Latino cultures (Hayes-Bautista and Chapa 1987; Klor de Alva 1988). However, the discussion that follows is based primarily on attitudes and behaviors of Latinos of Mexican origin.

There is a pervasive double standard with regard to attitudes toward sexual behavior for men and women. Women are expected not to show too much interest in sex, to be virgins at the time of their marriage, and to remain faithful to their husbands throughout marriage. Men, on the other hand, are expected to have an active sex life in order to live up to a cultural ideal of maleness. This double standard in terms of male and female sexual behavior has been noted in the Mexican culture (Carrier 1988; Espin 1984; Gonzalez Pineda 1972; Paz 1961; Peñalosa 1968) and in the Puerto Rican culture (Giraldo 1972). In the service of this cultural ideal, young boys are raised in an atmosphere that encourages them, through frequent joking and storytelling, to be highly sexualized and to seek multiple sexual outlets.

One of the sexual outlets sought by Mexican males is women who do not conform to the cultural ideal. These women are thought of as "bad" and are branded as prostitutes or "loose" women. However, the cost may be prohibitive for a man struggling with poverty to court a loose woman or to purchase the services of a prostitute. It has been speculated that, for this reason, a large number of Mexican males have turned to other males as sexual partners (Carrier 1976).

It is estimated that approximately 30% of Mexican males have engaged in sex with other men (Carrier 1985). The men who engage in this activity are not necessarily primarily sexually oriented toward other men and usually engage in heterosexual activities also. Researchers in this area have speculated that the high rate of bisexual behavior among Mexican males may be influenced by cultural beliefs that allow men to participate in certain sexual acts with other males without conceiving of themselves as homosexual. As long as the male engages in anal intercourse and assumes the active role of penetrator, he is not seen as a homosexual and does not risk any negative impact on his male image. Only the man who assumes the passive role and allows himself to be penetrated is considered homosexual (Carrier 1985; Magaña and Carrier, in press).

The fact that sex between men, consisting primarily of anal intercourse, is considered an acceptable sexual outlet and may be engaged in by nearly one-third of all Mexican men has vast implications for the spread of HIV. First, anal intercourse is one of the primary modes for transmission of the virus. Second, it is engaged in by individuals who do not consider themselves to be homosexual and therefore would not be receptive to AIDS education information targeted at that group. Perhaps the most alarming implication of this behavior pattern is that the men who engage in anal intercourse with large numbers of men also have sexual contact with women of childbearing age. This has added to the increase in HIV infection among Latino women and their children, who contract the disease from their infected mothers.

Sexual contact with prostitutes is another frequent sexual outlet for Latino men. This phenomenon has taken on some specific characteristics among Latinos in the United States that make it a particularly high-risk activity for the spread of HIV. In many areas of the United States where there are large numbers of undocumented Latino laborers, the prostitutes who offer their services to this population are most often intravenous-drug users (Blackmore et al. 1985; Magaña 1991; Rosenberg and Weiner 1988; M.A. Lawrence, A. Duque, L.M. Foster, J.R. Greenwood, unpublished data). These prostitutes usually have severe intravenous-drug use habits and have sexual relations with a large number of men, in rapid succession, in order to earn sufficient money to support their drug use habits.

Because intravenous-drug users have a very high rate of HIV infection, this activity also places the Latino population at high risk for contracting the disease. Again, the males who participate in sexual activity with intravenous-drug-using prostitutes are often also engaging in sexual contact with women of childbearing age.

Because of the dichotomy between the sexes and the double standard for male and female sexual behavior, it is culturally acceptable for the male to continue to pursue other sexual outlets after marriage. Because these sexual outlets often include the high-risk sexual activities discussed earlier in this chapter, the wife and unborn children are at an increased risk of contracting HIV.

## Working With Families of HIV-Infected Latino Children

In working with the families of HIV-infected Latino children, it is first important to assess who the significant members of the nuclear and extended family are. One of the basic differences between the Latino culture and the predominant United States culture is the pivotal role of the family in all aspects of life (Paz 1950; Peñalosa 1968). Typically, the Latino individual has close ties to members of the nuclear family as well as to members of the extended family. Often, several generations of the family live under one roof, and other members of the extended family, such as cousins, aunts, and uncles, may live together. If an individual has problems of any kind, he or she will usually turn to members of the extended family for support. If the family has been separated, as often happens when there has been a great deal of immigration and mobility in search of employment opportunities, Latinos will often rely heavily on fictive kinship networks such as the compadrazgo system—networks of close friends who become like family by virtue of being godparents to one another's children.

It is important for the health care professional to assess the family network of the pediatric AIDS patient. This is particularly important given the fact that usually both parents of the Latino pediatric patient are also infected. If they have not already, one or both of the child's parents may become ill and may die during the course of the child's illness. The health care professional must identify early who the supportive extended family members are, for these individuals will not only be pivotal in helping the parents cope with the child's illness, but they will most likely be the ones to take over the care of the child in the event of the parents' illness or death.

Education about HIV infection must be delivered to all members of the patient's social support system. The health care professional must remember the social and cultural factors that make it unlikely that Latino individuals have accurate knowledge regarding the AIDS virus. Information should be given to family members in Spanish (if that is their primary language) and in a manner that is consistent with the individual's level of educational attainment (Hochhauser 1987).

The health care professional will need to counsel the parents and family regarding the ultimate consequence of AIDS: death. Latino cultures experience death and dying very differently from Anglos (Kubler-Ross 1969; Shneidman 1984). Latino individuals are usually less reluctant to talk about death and tend to view it as just one more step in the cycle of life. Octavio Paz (1950), a well-known Mexican poet, has written about what he calls a Latino fascination with the topic of death and dying. He points out that death is often depicted in paintings, poems, and literature created by Latino individuals and that there are many indigenous groups in Mexico that celebrate the day of death with great festivities, as death is thought to represent the passing into a more pleasant phase in the cycle of life. It is perhaps this cultural fascination with death that often leads the AIDS patient of Mexican origin to overestimate the probability of his or her own death. It is important for health care professionals to ensure that these patients understand the difference between being HIV positive and having AIDS, because it is typical for the HIV-positive patient to assume that death is imminent. The distinction may need to be explained several times. It is often helpful for the health care professional to ask patients to explain their thoughts regarding the possibility of their eventual death and then to clarify misunderstandings.

Cultural attitudes toward death and dying among Latinos of Mexican origin probably make it easier for health care professionals to discuss openly the fact that death is the ultimate consequence of HIV infection. Latino families of Mexican origin will be less frightened and less prone to withdrawal and denial when this topic is raised than will Anglo families. However, as described above, sometimes the health care professional will see the opposite response. The patient may become obsessed with the prospect of death, and it becomes necessary to refocus his or her attention on planning for the remainder of life. For instance, mothers who are infected may focus attention exclusively on the task of arranging for their children's care and may neglect to make realistic plans for the time that they still have to spend together. The health care professional must be sensitive to these issues while helping the family plan for the child's care in the event of illness or death of one or both of the parents.

When working with pregnant HIV-infected Latino women, health care professionals need to be particularly sensitive to the discussion of abortion. The professional must be able to explain fully the possible health risks for the baby and to inform the woman of the availability of an abortion without conveying a preconceived notion of what the mother's response will be or should be. Some health care professionals may tend to convey a bias that all HIV-infected women should terminate their pregnancies, whereas others may convey an expectation that all Latino women are opposed to abortion because of their religious beliefs. In reality, some HIV-infected Latino women choose to have an abortion, whereas others choose to continue the pregnancy. The health care professional should be able to help the Latino woman reach her own decision and to support her regardless of what that decision is. In addition, because many Latino women are Catholic and the Catholic church opposes abortion, the health care professional must be particularly sensitive to the role of a woman's religious beliefs in her decision regarding whether to have an abortion and in her emotional adjustment once the decision has been made.

## Education and Prevention

It is important that AIDS education and prevention efforts take into account the socioeconomic, educational, and language characteristics of the Latino population. These efforts must also consider the unique cultural characteristics that determine attitudes and behaviors that have an effect on disease transmission and on the culture's receptiveness to various types of health education and prevention programs.

In general, health education and prevention programs aimed at reducing the spread of the AIDS virus in the Latino community must include aggressive outreach efforts so that the large numbers of Latinos who currently do not have access to health care can be reached. These services must be delivered in Spanish and must be culturally sensitive and appropriate for the educational status of the recipients.

Prevention programs designed to reduce the incidence of pediatric AIDS must be particularly sensitive to the cultural patterns of sexual behavior among Latinos. Given the subservient role of the Latino woman, it is difficult to come up with realistic strategies to help her protect herself (and her unborn children) from contracting HIV from a male partner. It might be suggested that Latino women be encouraged to use condoms as an exclusive means of birth control in order to simultaneously protect them from HIV infection. Although such a strategy might have some success in reducing HIV transmission, it might also result in an increase in unplanned pregnancies. Perhaps a more sound strategy would be for health care professionals to encourage the use of condoms in conjunction with another, more reliable form of birth control. Ultimately, to be most effective, prevention efforts must target the males whose high-risk sexual behavior is resulting in the increased incidence of HIV transmission to women and children. Given the high value placed on children and family in the Latino culture, perhaps the best way to motivate such men to change their behavior is to educate them regarding the possible consequences that their behavior may have for their yet-to-be-born children.

## Summary and Conclusions

Latinos make up a sizable and rapidly increasing proportion of the United States population, and they have been affected by HIV in a disproportionate manner. The high rates of HIV infection in the Latino population appear to be determined, at least in part, by two sets of complementary factors. The first set of factors consists of culturally determined sexual behaviors and beliefs that lead to a high risk for HIV transmission. Because these behaviors include high-risk sexual activities on the part of men who also have sexual relations with women of childbearing age, the incidence of HIV infection among women and children is also elevated.

The second set of factors that contribute to the high incidence of HIV infection in the Latino population has to do with the difficulty in delivering effective AIDS treatment and prevention services to this group. Because a large portion of the Latino population is living in poverty, many also without legal status in this country, access to health care is limited. Furthermore, the health education programs aimed at the general population are not likely to be effective with Latino groups due to language, educational, and cultural differences.

Services aimed at education, prevention, and treatment in the Latino community must be specially designed to fit the socioeconomic, language, and educational characteristics of the target group. Furthermore, if the groups most in need of services are to be accessed, health programs must include an aggressive outreach component that includes indigenous health promoters (Maduro 1983).

Prevention programs aimed at reducing the incidence of AIDS in Latino children must be sensitive to the cultural patterns of sexual behavior that can create a high risk for pediatric infection. To be most effective, prevention efforts should target the intravenous-drug-using Latino population, because it accounts for the majority of the Latino pediatric cases, but should not ignore Latino males whose high-risk sexual behavior appears to be a factor contributing to the increased incidence of HIV infection among Latino children.

# References

Bennet FJ: AIDS as a social phenomenon. Soc Sci Med 25(6):33–42, 1987

Blackmore CA, Limpakarnjanarat K, Rigsu-Perez JG, et al: An outbreak of chancroid in Orange County, California: descriptive epidemiology and disease-control measures. J Infect Dis 151(5):840–846, 1985

Carrier JM: Cultural factors affecting urban Mexican male homosexual behavior. Arch Sex Behav 5:103–124, 1976

Carrier JM: Mexican male bisexuality, in Bisexualities: Theory and Research. Edited by Klein F, Wolf T. New York, Haworth, 1985, pp 359–375

Carrier JM: Sexual behavior and spread of AIDS in Mexico. Med Anthropol 10(2–3):1–14, 1988

Centers for Disease Control: HIV/AIDS Surveillance Report. Atlanta, GA, Centers for Disease Control, 1991, pp 1–22

Chavez L: Settlers and sojourners: the case of Mexicans in the United States. Human Organization 47(2):95–108, 1988

Coates TJ, Temoshok L, Mandel J: Psychosocial research is essential to understanding and treating AIDS. Am Psychol 39(11):1309–1314, 1984

Cole M, Scribner S: Culture and Thought. New York, John Wiley, 1974

Espin OM: Cultural and historical influences on sexuality in Hispanic/Latin women: implications for psychotherapy, in Pleasure and Danger: Exploring Female Sexuality. Edited by Vance CS. Boston, MA, Routledge & Kegan Paul, 1984, pp 149–164

Giraldo O: El machismo como fenomeno psycocultural. Revista Latinoamericana de Psicologia 4(3):311–316, 1972

Gonzalez Pineda F: El Mexicano Psicologia de su Destructividad, 6th Edition. Mexico City, Mexico, Editorial Pax, 1972

Hanh R, Castro K: The health and health care status of Latino populations in the U.S.: a brief review. Paper presented at Latinos and AIDS: a National Strategy Symposium. Los Angeles, CA, February 1988

Hayes-Bautista D, Chapa J: Latino terminology: conceptual bases for standardized terminology. Am J Public Health 77:61–68, 1987

Hochhauser M: Readability of AIDS education materials. Paper presented at the 95th annual convention of the American Psychological Association, New York, December 1987

Kinnier RT: The need for psychosocial research on AIDS and counseling interventions for AIDS victims. Journal of Counseling and Development 64:472–481, 1986

Klor de Alva J: Telling Hispanics apart: Latino sociocultural diversity, in The Hispanic Experience in the United States. Edited by Acosta-Belen E, Sjostrom B. New York, Praeger, 1988, pp 41–61

Kubler-Ross E: On Death and Dying. New York, Macmillan, 1969

Maduro R: Curanderismo and Latino views of disease and curing. West J Med 139(6):64–70, 1983

Magaña JR: Sex, drugs and HIV: an ethnographic approach. Soc Sci Med 32(9):1–5, 1991

Magaña JR, Carrier JM: Mexican and Mexican American male sexual behavior and spreads of AIDS in California. Journal of Sex Research (in press)

Martin JL, Vance CS: Behavioral and psychosocial factors in AIDS: methodological and substantive issues. Am Psychol 39(11):1303–1312, 1984

McCarthy K, Burciaga R: Current and Future Effects of Mexican Immigration in California. Santa Monica, CA, Rand, 1988

Nelkin D: AIDS and the social sciences: review of useful knowledge and research needs. Rev Infect Dis 9:980–988, 1987

Nyamathi A, Vasquez R: Impact of poverty, homelessness, and drugs on Hispanic women at risk for HIV infection. Hispanic Journal of Behavioral Sciences 11:299–314, 1989

Paz O: The Labyrinth of Solitude: Life and Thought in Mexico. New York, Grove, 1961

Peñalosa F: Mexican family role. Journal of Marriage and Family 30:680–689, 1968

Rosenberg MJ, Weiner JM: Prostitutes and AIDS: a health department priority? Am J Public Health 78:418–423, 1988

Shneidman E (ed): Death: Current Perspectives. Mountain View, CA, Mayfield, 1984

Singer MC, Flores L, Davison G, et al: SIDA: the economic, social, and cultural context of AIDS among Latinos. Medical Anthropology Quarterly 4:72 107, 1990

Strategy Research Corporation: 1989 U.S. Hispanic Market. Miami, FL, Strategy Research Corporation, 1989

Chapter 4

# Adolescents

Mary Jane Rotheram-Borus, Ph.D.
Cheryl Koopman, Ph.D.

*T*he unique developmental characteristics of adolescents demand that clinical interventions and human immunodeficiency virus (HIV) prevention programs for adolescents be tailored quite differently from those for pediatric patients or adult patients (Hein 1989). The differences are reflected in the demographic profiles of infection, the structure of services delivered to youths, and the training that staff receive, as well as in the content, intensity, and impact of prevention messages. The goal of this chapter is to review these differences and outline the issues to be considered by those responsible for treating youths.

## HIV-Positive Adolescents

### *Epidemiology*

**Prevalence.** As of November 1989, 447 of the 115,158 cases of acquired immunodeficiency syndrome (AIDS) in the United States were diagnosed among adolescents 13–19 years of age (Centers for Disease Control 1989a). Although the prevalence of AIDS diagnosed among adolescents accounts for less than 1% of all cases of AIDS, this probably greatly underestimates the number of persons with AIDS who were infected during their adolescence, because the average incubation period

This work was supported by Grant 1P50 MH 43520 to the HIV Center for Clinical and Behavioral Studies from the National Institute of Mental Health and the National Institute on Drug Abuse, Anke Ehrhardt, Director. We appreciate the contributions of Clara Haignere, Donna Futterman, and Sten Vermund.

is over 10 years and 20% of AIDS cases have been diagnosed among adults aged 20–29 (Centers for Disease Control 1989a).

Although the number of adolescents infected with HIV is unknown, it is believed to be much higher than the number diagnosed with AIDS and is doubling each year (Brooks-Gunn et al. 1988). Among adolescents who are considered to be at high risk, seropositivity has ranged from 0.4% among Job Corps entrants (St. Louis et al. 1989) and emergency room and adolescent clinic users (D'Angelo et al. 1989), to 1% of all females under 19 giving birth in New York City public hospitals (New York City Health Department 1990), to 2.2% of those attending clinics for sexually transmitted diseases (Quinn et al. 1988), to 6.7% of runaways (Stricof et al. 1988). Also, because high-risk behaviors such as sex and drug use are typically initiated during adolescence, many uninfected youths are at risk of becoming infected due to their behavior.

**Gender and ethnic differences.**    Prevalence and routes of HIV infection differ by gender and ethnicity. Among adolescents, the percentage of females with AIDS (18%) is greater than that among adults (9%; Centers for Disease Control 1989b). Female adolescents with AIDS are much more likely to have become infected through heterosexual activity (41%) than are male adolescents with AIDS (2%; Centers for Disease Control 1989c). In contrast, among male adolescents with AIDS, 38% of cases are associated with homosexual activity and 37% with hemophilia, a pattern also reflected in the large urban epicenters (Centers for Disease Control 1989c). In a blind seroprevalence study of 3,124 blood specimens of urban adolescents, the seropositivity rate was found to be higher among females (0.5%) than among males (0.2%; D'Angelo et al. 1989). One reason for greater risk to female adolescents is that the higher ratio of infected males to infected females results in more heterosexual females than males having infected partners (Hearst and Hulley 1988). Another reason is that female adolescents tend to have sexual relations with males who are several years older, who are more likely to be HIV infected.

There are also important ethnic differences among adolescents. AIDS is more common among black and Hispanic adolescents than among white adolescents (Centers for Disease Control 1989a). For example, the Job Corps seroprevalence data show that among 17-year-old males, the seroprevalence rate was over three times greater among blacks than among whites (Hayman and St. Louis 1989). Among adolescents, the risk factors most associated with HIV transmission differ considerably across ethnicity: for example, among adolescents with AIDS, blacks are more likely than whites or Hispanics to have engaged in homosexual activity, and Hispanics are more likely than blacks or whites to have used intravenous drugs (Centers for Disease Control 1989c). Among adolescent Hispanics, the risk factors also vary by geographic region. Most Hispanic adolescent AIDS cases in Puerto Rico and northern U.S. states are due to intravenous-drug use and heterosexual relations, whereas in Florida, Texas, and California, homosexual relations is the major risk factor (Castro and Manoff 1988).

**Disease progression.** There are few systematic data about how adolescents with AIDS differ from adults or children with AIDS in disease progression, except for individuals with hemophilia. Among hemophilia patients who are seropositive, adolescents and children remain disease free significantly longer than do adults (Goeddert et al. 1990). However, data on patients with hemophilia are not likely to generalize to adolescents who have become infected through high-risk sexual and drug use behavior. When adolescents are experiencing multiple problems (e.g., poverty or homelessness, use of nonintravenous drugs, sexual abuse, and HIV seropositivity), the course of infection may be quite different.

Information is lacking about the effectiveness of drugs to treat HIV-positive adolescents. Until recently, adolescents ages 13–18 years were excluded from clinical trials testing the effectiveness of drugs such as zidovudine (AZT) and Bactrim to prevent Pneumocystis carinii pneumonia; however, clinical trials with adolescents are now ongoing.

Clinicians also lack adequate information to tailor the dosage of such medications for particular adolescents. Recommended dosages are often geared to the average adult-size male, without including specific instructions on how to adapt them to the needs of others such as small adolescent females.

Furthermore, the clinician needs to consider the adolescent's cognitive development in attempting to establish a treatment regimen. Adolescents, even more than adults, may lack the ability to understand why they should take medication when they feel healthy and have not experienced disease symptoms. The sense of invulnerability that characterizes many adolescents also plays a role in reducing their motivation to comply with medical treatment.

## Intervention

Interventions for seropositive adolescents can emphasize goals at the individual level—for example, to help HIV-positive adolescents to stay healthy—and at the public health level—for example, to avoid infecting others. In promoting health at the individual level, interventions differ according to the needs of the individual: 1) providing HIV testing to determine serostatus to youth engaging in high-risk behavior, 2) following asymptomatic seropositive adolescents to provide services tailored to their health status, and 3) providing clinical services to adolescents sick with AIDS. These interventions also have public health implications that sometimes conflict with the needs of individual adolescents, forcing clinicians to make difficult decisions.

**Considerations regarding HIV testing of adolescents.**   There is controversy about when it is appropriate to provide HIV testing to adolescents. Those youths who are most likely to be seropositive due to their high-risk behaviors often have other characteristics that undermine the benefits of informing them of their serostatus. A decision to initiate testing assumes that if persons know their serostatus they will then have access to prophylactic treatments (e.g., AZT), monitor their health status, seek health services, and be motivated to change their high-risk behaviors. Only under these circumstances is testing useful. Developmentally, adolescents are not characterized by such responsible, mature, and altruistic behavior, nor do they typically have independent access to health services. Adolescents must understand the consequences of HIV testing before it is initiated.

Because poor minority youths are overrepresented among the HIV-positive group, there are serious, long-term potential outcomes of being informed of their serostatus. For homeless youths under the supervision of the Department of Social Services, HIV positivity can exclude youths from receiving services from most group home and shelter care systems in most cities. Jobs and insurance may be much more difficult to secure, and substantial energy must be expended to obtain health services.

However, it is not clear that evaluators can assess adolescents' competence to understand these consequences in one hour, the typical period allotted to pretest counseling. Prerequisites for understanding the consequences of HIV testing may be interpersonal problem-solving ability and formal operational thought. Many adolescents have not acquired the ability to think abstractly and to consider several alternatives simultaneously by the age of 18. Those youths who may be most at risk are also those most likely to have deficits in these skills. For example, 30% of New York City homeless youths, the adolescents with the highest known seropositivity rate (6.7%; Stricof et al. 1988), have attempted suicide in the past (Shaffer and Caton 1984). Individuals who attempt suicide have poor interpersonal problem-solving ability. Furthermore, past suicidal behavior is the best predictor of future suicidal behavior (Trautman and Shaffer 1984). It may be unwise to provide HIV testing to youths with histories of suicide attempts, because the suicide rate has been reported to be 36 times higher among persons with AIDS (Marzuk et al. 1988).

Potential suicidal behavior is not the only concern making public health officials hesitant to test adolescents. Many youths whose behaviors place them at highest risk for HIV infection have a history of behavior problems and antisocial acts. An epidemiological study of runaway youth suggests that 72% of male runaways and 55% of female runaways meet criteria for a diagnosis of conduct disorder (Shaffer and Caton 1984). Adolescents who often engage in antisocial acts might well use sexual intercourse as a lethal weapon to express angry feelings. Should a diagnosis of conduct disorder lead to the decision to exclude a young person from HIV testing? When youths with conduct problems or a history of suicidality learn that they are HIV positive, mental health services are likely to be necessary to help them with potential depression and violent fantasies.

Finally, parental rights to demand and be informed regarding the outcome of HIV testing present a thorny ethical issue. The rights of the youth to receive testing, as well as information about sex and drugs, often need to be considered against the rights of the parents to restrict such exposure. At question is whether youths have rights to information so that they can modify their behavior to protect themselves, or whether youths do not have such rights because they are under the protection of their parents and communities that have the responsibility for guiding sexual behavior. In Kentucky, recent legislation gives courts and social service agencies the right to demand HIV testing of adolescents (English 1987), a right that many service providers have been hesitant to help exercise. These are difficult ethical dilemmas and complex clinical decisions. Thus, HIV testing and pretest counseling for adolescents may demand far more extensive assessment, staff training, and planning for the follow-up clinical care and services than may be required for other risk groups.

**Serving HIV-positive youths.** Few clinical programs are specifically tailored for adolescents; thus, adolescents are often channeled into programs designed for adults or children. This is particularly true in infectious disease clinics, where the HIV-seropositive patient is likely to be treated. Because the number of adolescent AIDS cases is relatively low, almost all of these clinics have been designed primarily for adults. The number of such clinics has grown exponentially over the last few years. The caseloads of health workers are typically overwhelming, the services are characterized by the requirement of extensive bureaucratic paperwork before help can be received, and the clinics are typically hospital based, commonly isolated from the community.

In large urban centers, there are a few positive models of services that have been designed for HIV-positive youths (e.g., Montefiore Medical Center, New York City; Children's Hospital, Los Angeles; University of Washington, Seattle) that share a number of characteristics. First, case recruitment and referral and patient management are recognized as requiring community-based networks of service providers. For example, in New York City, HIV-positive youths often have contact with several social service agencies (a runaway shelter, an adolescent drop-in center, a hospital-based clinic, and an alternative school). However, no single agency may know the full details of the adolescent's background, current living situation, or health status. Information and coordination of information and services are typically necessary to provide good clinical care. Without a service delivery network, several different hospitals may conduct complete health workups, duplicating others' work. Therefore, in New York City an Adolescent AIDS Network helps service providers to develop administrative protocols to facilitate sharing of information, without violating youths' rights to confidentiality. Such networks also help agencies to develop services that complement those already provided in the community, rather than duplicating services.

Medical services are only the tip of the iceberg for services required by HIV-positive youth. These youths are also likely to need housing, psychotherapy, and social, educational, legal, and financial help. Given the variety of services that will be required on an ongoing basis by an HIV-positive youth, it is critical that a case manager coordinate services across agencies. Perhaps most important, networks foster personal relationships among service providers, the most effective link needed to secure speedy and responsive health care for adolescents.

Second, adolescents are not motivated to seek treatment and will not go unless the atmosphere is inviting, humane, and nonbureaucratic (with minimum red tape). This requires that services be structured in consideration of adolescents' developmental characteristics, with staff who understand these developmental features. All staff members who work with HIV-positive patients must be provided with basic knowledge about AIDS, routine medical safety procedures, issues of death and dying, and community resources. In addition, staff must be prepared to be "tested" by adolescents—the staff must set limits in a consistent fashion with youths without losing their temper when adolescents repeatedly violate agency rules. Deciding when to refer a youth to a different agency and knowing the appropriate referral are difficult choices. Adolescents often do not recognize their own best interests; therefore, staff need to be prepared for adolescents to behave self-destructively, such as disclosing their serostatus to persons who may use it to discriminate against them. Finally, youths who are most likely to be HIV positive may also have problematic relationships with their parents, have a history of sexual and/or physical abuse or neglect, and engage in other risk behaviors (Rotheram-Borus et al. 1989a). Thus, staff may need extensive preparation for ethical issues they may encounter and for establishing referral and treatment resources for these special problems. Training that empowers staff and adolescents in each of these areas is critical for designing services for HIV-positive youths.

Because adolescents do not have the rights of adults, two specific issues arise. Disenfranchised, HIV-positive adolescents need help in obtaining AZT, which can cost thousands of dollars, an amount far beyond the means of these adolescents and their families. Also, although there are laws against discrimination based on serostatus, HIV-positive youths may need legal help and counseling specifically to protect their rights to receive education and other benefits.

Finally, comprehensive care will be necessary to maintain the health of HIV-positive adolescents and to help them avoid high-risk behaviors. They need health checkups once every 6 months and as they become symptomatic even more frequently. The positive mental health response and resiliency of the adult gay community to HIV has been seen as unique (Rabkin 1989). It is not clear that there is such a reaction among youths. In fact, clinicians report the opposite. It can be anticipated that mental health services for follow-up counseling to reduce risk behaviors will frequently be necessary among HIV-positive youths. Because youths who are most likely to become HIV positive are those who engage in multiple risk behaviors, psychotherapeutic interventions, particularly with adolescents in therapeutic supportive groups, need to be provided by the psychiatric community.

## Prevention Among Youths Engaging in High-Risk Sexual and Drug Use Behaviors

### *Epidemiology of Risk Behaviors*

**Unprotected sexual acts.**  Most adolescents are sexually active by the time they are 18 years old, although the estimates vary according to the population examined, with the average age at onset of sexual activity varying by gender and ethnicity (Zelnick and Kantner 1980). Ninety percent of the 16-year-olds from blue-collar families in a recent study in the Midwest reported sexual experience (Orr et al. 1989). Further risk for HIV infection through sexual transmission comes from the experimentation with multiple partners that is typical of many adolescents (Zelnick and Kantner 1980). Adolescents engaging in "survival sex"—an exchange of sex for money, shelter, or drugs—also increase their risk because under such conditions they are more likely to engage in high-risk sex with persons of unknown HIV status.

Adolescents are also unlikely to consistently use condoms or other methods of protection that could reduce their chances of infection. Reports of consistent condom use among adolescents range from 2% to 10% of the females and 0 to 8% of the males coming to health clinics in Little Rock, Baltimore, or San Francisco (Kegeles et al. 1988; Rickert et al. 1989; Seifert-McLean 1989) to 23% of the males and 14% of the females among secondary students (Otis et al. 1989). The severity of the threat of unprotected sexual intercourse is underscored by pregnancies among 33% of all sexually active unmarried adolescent females (Zelnick and Kantner 1980) and over 200,000 cases of gonorrhea among adolescents annually (Centers for Disease Control 1988a). Although females are dependent on cooperation by male sexual partners in use of condoms, female adolescents perceive the need to convince their sexual partners to use condoms as a major barrier to condom use (Otis et al. 1989).

**Substance abuse.** Experimentation with drugs, another activity associated with increased risk for HIV infection, is typically initiated during adolescence. Few adolescents inject drugs intravenously, a risk behavior for HIV infection because of the likelihood of sharing needles or works with infected persons. In recent surveys, the percentages of high school students who had intravenously injected drugs ranged from 2.8% in Michigan to 4.1% in California to 6.3% in Washington, D.C., although typically males were more likely than females to have used intravenous drugs (Centers for Disease Control 1988b).

Far greater numbers of adolescents use drugs without injecting them, such as smoking marijuana or hashish. Recent surveys of high school seniors found that 93% had used alcohol, 59% had smoked marijuana, and 16% had used cocaine (Clayton and Voss 1982). Abuse of these substances increases risk for HIV infection in two ways. First, use of these drugs can operate as a "gateway" to intravenous use of heroin or cocaine. Adolescents are unrealistically confident regarding their ability to experiment with drugs without becoming hooked on addictive substances. Second, the high levels of abuse of alcohol and nonintravenous drugs lower adolescents' inhibitions for unsafe sexual behavior.

**Knowledge of and attitudes toward HIV.** In the United States, adolescents appear to have a moderately high level of knowledge of AIDS (demonstrating about 75–80% accurate knowledge). A high level of knowledge about AIDS does not appear to keep adolescents from engaging in risk behavior. In terms of general knowledge, young people know about the connection between AIDS and death. However, youths do not personalize this knowledge to perceive themselves as being at risk for AIDS. The effectiveness of fear tactics to personalize knowledge of the association between sex and AIDS has been demonstrated (Rhodes et al. 1989); however, it is unclear how increasing youths' fears related to their sexuality would affect their normal sexual development.

Adolescents evaluate themselves unrealistically as competent to implement safe behaviors. Their self-reports of being capable of implementing safe behaviors are contradicted by their behavior reported in epidemiological surveys. For example, in focus groups, many youths are incapable even in simulated role-plays of implementing these behaviors. Often, their reported sexual behavior contradicted their assertions of being capable of acting safely (Rotheram-Borus et al. 1989a).

So far, it appears that adolescents' behavior change in response to the AIDS epidemic has been minimal. In a telephone survey of 656 adolescents (Strunin and Hingson 1987), only 3% of the total reported that they had changed their behavior in response to the epidemic in ways believed to reduce their chances of infection (e.g., abstinence or condom use). Programs of two to three sessions emphasizing education (Di-Clemente et al. 1989) and of three sessions of behavioral rehearsals (Kipke et al. 1989) have not demonstrated behavior change.

## Prerequisites for Successful Prevention

To change their high-risk behaviors, adolescents need intensive programs that encourage behavioral strategies known to reduce risk for HIV infection. However, all available strategies are controversial, including abstinence, monogamy, screening partners, HIV testing, and explicit instruction in sterilizing needles and hypodermic syringes and safer sex practices (Rotheram-Borus and Koopman 1991). To encourage any of these behavioral strategies, four components of AIDS prevention need to be addressed (Kelly et al. 1989): general knowledge, personalized knowledge, social competence, and access to resources. The effectiveness of programs emphasizing these components has been demonstrated for gay adult males (Kelly et al. 1989) and high-risk adolescents (Rotheram-Borus et al. 1989b).

**General knowledge about AIDS and HIV.**   Adolescents need to have general knowledge about HIV and AIDS as a prerequisite to safer behavior. Six domains of general knowledge of AIDS have been identified: definitions, outcomes of HIV infection and AIDS, risk behavior, routes of transmission, prevention methods, and HIV testing (Koopman et al. 1990). Although being informed about HIV and AIDS is thought to be an important basis for guiding safer behavior, general knowledge is insufficient for promoting behavior change. Even among adult gay males, although knowledge does appear to be one prerequisite, it is not sufficient for reducing high-risk behavior (Stall et al. 1988). Therefore, other foundations of safer behavior need to be addressed.

**Personalized knowledge of AIDS.**   This involves the application of general knowledge of AIDS to one's own situation. The Health Belief Model suggests that personalized knowledge is a prerequisite for motivating adolescents toward safer behavior (Janz and Becker 1984). Three domains of personalized knowledge have been identified: 1) response efficacy—a belief that AIDS can be prevented, 2) self-efficacy—a belief in one's personal competency to act safely, and 3) a perceived threat of HIV infection. Research conducted with high-risk adolescents in New York City has found that this personalized knowledge about AIDS is significantly associated with safer sexual behavior (Rotheram-Borus et al. 1989c). Positive attitudes and beliefs about AIDS prevention build on adolescents' knowledge of AIDS.

A variety of attitudes and beliefs have been identified that may be relevant to implementing safe acts (DiClemente et al. 1986; Koopman et al. 1990). For example, two important beliefs are that one's peers support safe acts and that one has self-control over one's behavior. Also of potential relevance to behavior is the expectation that one will act to prevent pregnancy.

**Social competence.** To implement safer acts, adolescents need to be socially competent. For example, adolescents need to be able to handle being teased by their peers for refusing to engage in unsafe acts. The intensity of adolescents' concern about others' reactions to their behavior is demonstrated by the level of embarrassment they report about buying condoms (Gladis et al. 1989). Thus, adolescents need to be able to refuse to engage in sexual intercourse, to request that a condom be used during sexual intercourse, and to negotiate substituting safer acts for high-risk acts. The importance of social competence is suggested by the effectiveness of programs targeting risk-reduction behaviors among adult gay males that have emphasized the development of social competence (Kelly et al. 1989; Valdiserri et al. 1989).

Empirically based models of social competence are needed that are tailored to the norms of specific cultural and ethnic groups to develop youths' social skills, enabling them to substitute safe acts for high-risk acts. For example, there is little awareness of how a socially competent Mexican-American girl's refusal of her boyfriend might be quite different from that of her black female peer. It is less challenging to cultural identity and probably more effective in producing behavior change when persons designing programs are aware of and sensitive to differences in youths' cultural norms. In particular there is a need for researchers to identify norms of social competence on which to base the design of interventions congruent with youths' cultural backgrounds.

**Access to resources.**    Knowledge of AIDS and intending to act safely are useless without access to resources (e.g., condoms available 24 hours a day), including comprehensive health care. Youths' high-risk behavior may be the result of attempting to cope with an environment that undermines their feeling lovable and competent and other aspects of self-esteem and security. For example, adolescents who lack the security of feeling that they have adequate access to resources may be more likely to engage in survival sex. Therefore, to reduce risky behavior, the environment needs to be consciously restructured as a holistic system for meeting youths' needs, including furnishing support for managing difficult external events (e.g., eviction from home, sexually transmitted diseases, unplanned pregnancy, legal problems).

**Delivery model.**    Behavioral engineering is critical to the design of programs for adolescents that address the four components outlined above (general and personalized knowledge of AIDS, social competence, and access to resources). This means that programs must be fun and rewarding, build on youths' strengths rather than target deficits, mobilize peer support, provide positive and realistic role models, and be consistent with the norms and values of the community and the setting in which they are delivered. One component that has been largely ignored is family involvement in both the design and implementation of interventions. Far greater attention must be paid to involving families, especially when the cultural and ethnic background of the youth being served is different from that of those delivering the intervention.

Addressing these components requires that interventions be more intensive than the 2–3 hours typically allotted in schools (DiClemente et al. 1989). In our own program, we believed that a 10-hour program was perhaps the minimum length necessary to feasibly hope for behavior change and the maximum length that could feasibly be replicated in other settings. Preliminary results from the 10-hour program indicate positive behavior changes, particularly with increased condom use (Rotheram-Borus et al. 1989b). However, because some youths received more than 30 sessions, we found that the more exposure youths had to the program, the greater the behavior change ($r = .52$; Rotheram-Borus et al. 1989b).

The format of the program requires considerable attention. Youth do not want to sit in groups and learn about HIV. Knowledge about AIDS is typically acquired in our program in video workshops where youths design posters, public service announcements, and raps about AIDS or make brief dramatizations of high-risk situations. Personalizing risk is addressed by having each individual build a risk hierarchy, a scale from 0 to 100 where youths identify situations of low-, medium-, and high-risk situations for themselves. Socially competent and safe acts in these risk situations are then rehearsed in both same-sex and mixed-sex groups so that youths feel comfortable in implementing safe acts. Youths are exposed to babies in orphanages and see HIV-infected babies and persons with AIDS to enhance their perceived threat of HIV. Each group session begins with youths bragging about successes in acting safely with their peers. Although there are many good AIDS prevention training manuals, selection should be based on reviewing whether such programs involve basic principles of behavior change, peers' support, and intensive intervention. The Centers for Disease Control can provide a review of videos and training manuals for adolescents.

## Issues Critical to Providing Good Clinical Care

### Background Risk Factors

**Sexual abuse.** There is uncertainty regarding the precise prevalence of sexual abuse in the general population of adolescents, due to differences in samples, measures, and procedures used in the research. Rates of sexual abuse have been reported ranging from 6% to 62% for females and from 3% to 31% for males (Peters et al. 1986). In some populations, such as homeless youth, sexual abuse may be so common that a major component of AIDS prevention efforts may need to focus on addressing issues of sexual abuse. Even the smaller prevalence estimates justify considering the issue of sexual abuse in efforts to prevent HIV infection among adolescents. Because AIDS prevention involves explicit discussion of sexuality, it must be anticipated that those who have been abused may have strong emotional reactions to prevention efforts.

Substantial research has shown that for many years after the sexual abuse, and sometimes for decades, sexual abuse can impair the victim's functioning and lead to depression, suicide attempts, dissociation, and interpersonal disturbances (Browne and Finkelhor 1986). Furthermore, of particular concern for AIDS prevention efforts, sexual abuse is often associated with a compulsive desire for sex (Browne and Finkelhor 1986), which may lead the sexually abused adolescent to engage in high-risk sexual activities or sex with many partners (Rotheram-Borus et al. 1989a).

When conducting AIDS prevention programs or research with adolescents, several guidelines must be considered (Rotheram-Borus et al. 1989a): 1) The highly sensitive nature of sexual abuse requires that disclosure of this topic must be conducted only in personal interviews to protect the adolescent's privacy. 2) Questions about past sexual history may elicit more accurate reports if the adolescent is asked about uninvited or upsetting or unwanted sexual experiences than about being forced to have sex. 3) Before inquiring about sexual abuse, trained and experienced clinicians must be available to provide help if needed when painful emotions are elicited. 4) It is important to acknowledge sexual abuse in general group discussions of sexuality, for example, to say, "Many of you in this group may have experienced uninvited sexual acts and have strong feelings about how this may affect your relationship with other persons."

**Sexual orientation.**    Among adolescents, the prevalence of homosexual activity is not known, as there are few recent data. The available data from a 1948 study by Kinsey et al. showed high rates of homosexual behavior among males (48% of 15-year-olds and 37% of 18-year-olds). Seventy percent of all persons who are HIV infected are gay males, and because 10% of all gay males with AIDS are in their 20s (Owen 1985), many were probably infected during their teens. Sexual partners of adolescent gay males tend to be much older on average (Remafedi 1987), and adult gay males are a population that is at high risk for HIV infection. Furthermore, unprotected anal intercourse, frequently practiced among gay males who have not changed their sexual practices, is a high-risk sexual behavior.

In contrast to males, homosexual activity by females does not appear to be a common route for HIV infection; however, given the high rates of bisexual activity that we have found among gay male adolescents in New York City, bisexual female adolescents may be at high risk for HIV infection if the social networks from which they draw male sexual partners include a high concentration of bisexual males.

Services to help gay adolescents must help them with a variety of stressors that may influence their ability to behave safely and protect their health. Stressors faced by gay adolescents include others' anticipated negative reactions to self-disclosure of their gay identity and fears of rejection by their families and communities if their sexual orientation is discovered (Rotheram-Borus et al. 1991). Also, gay adolescents are vulnerable to violent attacks by biased persons, which continue to be widespread (Hunter 1989). The limited social networks of gay adolescents may leave them feeling isolated due to their sexual orientation, less able to manage the additional stressors they encounter.

**Psychosexual milestones.** For those youths who have not initiated sexual intercourse, prevention efforts are typically directed at delaying the onset of sexual intercourse. Programs to reduce smoking and alcohol use and to increase healthy eating habits have consistently found that it is much harder to change existing habits than it is to delay the development of a habit (Hayes 1987). White females' sexual development typically follows a sequence (e.g., first holding hands, then kissing, then breast fondling, then genital petting, and, finally, intercourse). This sequence suggests that for these girls there may be several opportunities within this sequence to encourage youths to proceed more slowly through these milestones, thus delaying the onset of sexual intercourse.

However, cultural norms regarding sexuality are relevant when considering alternatives to high-risk sexual behavior. Black females do not typically proceed along the same route of sexual milestones as do white females; they engage in sexual intercourse at earlier ages, often before they have experienced other sexual milestones (Hayes 1987). For example, among some black adolescents, holding hands or petting may have rarely, if ever, occurred, even though they engage in sexual intercourse (Rotheram-Borus et al. 1989a). Thus, encouraging black adolescents to engage in psychosexual milestones other than intercourse may affect their ethnic identity (Rotheram-Borus et al. 1989a). Furthermore, low-risk sexual activities, such as genital petting, are valued differently by various cultures. In our own prevention program, such concerns have led us to mention kissing, hand-holding, and petting as alternatives that some people may choose as safe ways of expressing affection, while neither encouraging nor discouraging youth from engaging in these activities.

**Adolescents with multiple behavior problems.** Risk behaviors tend to cluster within individuals. Adolescents at high risk for HIV infection due to sexual acts or intravenous-drug use are also likely to be depressed and anxious, to have low self-esteem, to be more likely to attempt suicide, to abuse nonintravenous drugs and alcohol, and to have a history of antisocial behavior leading to trouble with the law and at school (Ensminger, in press). The psychological distress associated with these problems is likely to mediate adolescents' risk-taking behavior. Distressed youths are more likely to engage in high-risk sex or drug use behavior to alleviate unpleasant mood states, increasing their chances of becoming infected with HIV. It is because of this clustering that services for adolescents must be comprehensive, addressing a variety of adolescent problems.

For example, runaway youths are perceived as being a group frequently engaging in this multiple-risk-behavior pattern (Shaffer and Caton 1984), and the seropositivity rate among this group confirms the concern (6.7%; Stricof et al. 1988). According to a 1985 survey of programs for runaway and homeless youth, 62% of the respondents stated that the youths who they were serving appear to have more problems than the youths 5 or 6 years previously (Children's Defense Fund 1988). Another study found that over 40% of the Ohio children in foster care placement had multiple problems (Children in Out-of-Home Care, cited in Children's Defense Fund 1988). Furthermore, these behaviors seem to be associated with stressful life events; runaway youth appear to have four times the number of stressful events in the last 3 months compared with other groups of youth: 16% have been assaulted, 55% have had trouble at school, 24% have been pregnant, 22% have had contact with the police, and 20% have been sexually abused (Rotheram-Borus et al. 1991). AIDS prevention must address these other problems. Why would an adolescent who did not have plans for his or her next meal or bed care about safe sex?

## Assessing Risk Behaviors

**Anticipated problems.** Given that adolescents are likely to be at considerable risk for HIV infection, clinicians need to be able to assess their risk behaviors. Several methodological problems have been identified in research on youth at risk that need to be dealt with when trying to evaluate youths' risk:

1. *Unrealistic expectations* (Rotheram-Borus et al. 1989a). Youths often report that they expect to date for several months, fall in love, and discuss supporting each other before they become sexually involved. These expectations are not supported by reports of their past behavior,

which indicate that they have had more than one partner in the last 3 months and have never discussed their relationship. When interviewing youths about their behavior and plans, a strategy to help youths identify and confront their unrealistic expectations is to ask youths to concretely role-play or demonstrate their plans for implementing safe acts. For example, the clinician may ask an adolescent girl to role-play how she would handle an encounter when an attractive older boy invites her to use cocaine or how to ask the boy to use a condom. One technique particularly useful in simulating the realistic context of high-risk encounters is to ask youths to stand facing each other, 6 inches apart, while role-playing. Being able to sustain assertiveness when being touched is a central issue affecting youths' ability to implement safe acts. It is important for the clinician to make all simulations as realistic as possible for youths.

2. *Inconsistency across reporting methods* (Sandberg et al. 1988) *and underreporting.* The clinician can use a battery of assessment techniques that includes personal interviews, clinical notes of observations, and questionnaires. To help youths to feel comfortable, it may help to normalize atypical responses by creating a nonjudgmental atmosphere. One strategy for creating such an atmosphere is to ask open-ended, lengthy questions containing many words. This has been found to increase respondents' willingness to report sensitive information about alcohol use and sex (Blair et al. 1977) and may increase the reporting of drug use, as well. Another strategy is to encourage reporting of atypical behavior by using a tone of voice conveying that it is not atypical, that the behavior was expected, or to provide false information about the prevalence of an act. For example, a clinician may query, "When was the last time you engaged in group sex?" Ethical concerns discourage these strategies, particularly in research settings. There are, however, innovative strategies for increasing honest disclosures in research settings. For example, the randomized response technique involves simultaneously asking sensitive and innocuous questions where the answers are not reported in the order asked, for example, "Have you used intravenous drugs, and is your mother's birthday in July?" Base rates of risk behaviors can be calculated from responses to the questions without youths disclosing their personal risk behavior.

3. *Failure to understand terms and questions.* Those who address sexuality and substance abuse among adolescents must be comfortable discussing these issues. It is critical to provide sensitization training to

all clinical staff involved in assessment and intervention with youths. This training includes being comfortable with slang words for sexual acts, which may be the only terms understood by youths (e.g., "cunt" for a vagina), and with discussing sexual acts and strategies to cope in high-risk situations.

## Summary

The clinician has a dual role to play in helping adolescents regarding HIV and AIDS, both in daily practice and in advocating for societal changes. In daily practice, the clinician must keep in mind the different needs of three groups of adolescents—those diagnosed with AIDS, those HIV positive, and those uninfected engaging in high-risk behaviors. For those diagnosed with AIDS, clinicians will need to establish access to services, tailor services to adolescents' needs, and consider the parent or guardian's rights and responsibilities for deciding care. For adolescents who may be HIV positive, clinicians will need to consider whether HIV testing is likely to result in greater harm than good (e.g., if the youth may be suicidal) and to establish access to follow-up services for those adolescents who receive HIV testing. For uninfected adolescents engaging in high-risk behavior, clinicians need to decide which prevention strategies to recommend and to provide intervention that promotes general knowledge, personalized knowledge, social competence, and access to supportive services, while considering background risk factors.

There are a number of societal changes that clinicians can advocate regarding HIV and AIDS to benefit adolescents. Clinicians are in credible situations to advocate for more treatment programs for drug addicts, who are in danger of transmitting HIV through pregnancy and breast-feeding of infants as well as through needle sharing and sexual acts. To help adolescents who have AIDS or who are HIV positive, clinicians can help to educate the public about the inadequacy of medical care available to adolescents and advocate for access to AZT and other medicines that are proven to prolong life for HIV-positive persons. Because little research has been done on the effects of AZT and other medications to help adolescents in particular, another way to help is to encourage the funding of medical research targeting adolescents.

For helping to reduce risk behaviors of adolescents, an important societal change that clinicians can advocate is to provide adolescents with attractive role models deriving satisfaction from safe behavior. This draws from social learning theory, asserting that the behavior intended to supplant the high-risk behavior (e.g., condom use during intercourse) must be associated with powerful reinforcers. Clinicians can urge that societal messages about sex and drugs for adolescents show highly attractive role models demonstrating how satisfaction can result from safe behavior. In a parallel campaign to prevent drunk driving (Rothenberg 1990), weekly programs have shown their lead actors refraining from drinking alcohol when driving ("No thanks, I'm the designated driver"). The threat that AIDS poses to adolescents necessitates experimenting with new approaches for helping adolescents manage risk behaviors that are difficult to change.

## References

Blair E, Sudman S, Bradburn NM, et al: How to ask questions about drinking and sex: response effects in measuring consumer behavior. Journal of Marketing Research 14:316–321, 1977

Brooks-Gunn J, Boyer CB, Hein K: Preventing HIV infection and AIDS in children and adolescents: behavioral research and intervention strategies. Am Psychol 43:958–964, 1988

Browne A, Finkelhor D: Initial and longterm effects: a review of the research, in Sourcebook on Child Sexual Abuse. Edited by Finkelhor D, Araji S, Baron L, et al. Beverly Hills, CA, Sage, 1986, pp 143–179

Castro KG, Manoff SB: The epidemiology of AIDS in Hispanic adolescents, in The AIDS Challenge: Prevention Education for Young People. Edited by Quackenbush M, Nelson M, Clark K. Santa Cruz, CA, Network Publications, 1988, pp 321–333

Centers for Disease Control: Sexually transmitted diseases: statistics for 1987. Atlanta, GA, Centers for Disease Control, 1988a

Centers for Disease Control: HIV related beliefs, knowledge and behavior among high school students. MMWR 35:421–424, 1988b

Centers for Disease Control: AIDS cases reported through November 1989: HIV/AIDS surveillance. Atlanta, GA, Centers for Disease Control, December 1989a

Centers for Disease Control: Adolescent (13–19 year old) AIDS: sex and transmission category: United States through 12/31/88 (slide). Atlanta, GA, Centers for Disease Control, 1989b

Centers for Disease Control: Adolescent (13–19 year old) AIDS: transmission category and race/ethnicity: United States through 12/31/88 (slide). Atlanta, GA, Centers for Disease Control, 1989c

Children's Defense Fund: A children's defense budget FY 1989: an analysis of our nation's investment in children. Washington, DC, Children's Defense Fund, 1988

Clayton RR, Voss HL: Technical review on drug abuse and dropouts. Rockville, MD, National Institute on Drug Abuse, 1982, pp 1–44

D'Angelo LJ, Getson P, Luban N, et al: HIV infection in adolescents: can we predict who is at risk, in Abstracts of the 5th International Conference on AIDS. Ottawa, Ontario, Canada, International Research Development Center, 1989, p 712

DiClemente RJ, Zorn J, Temoshok L: Adolescents and AIDS: a survey of knowledge, beliefs and attitudes about AIDS in San Francisco. Am J Public Health 76:1443–1445, 1986

DiClemente RJ, Pies CA, Stoller EJ, et al: Evaluation of school-based AIDS education curricula in San Francisco. Journal of Sex Research 26:188–198, 1989

English A: Adolescents and AIDS: legal and ethical questions multiply. Youth Law News 8(6):1–6, 1987

Ensminger ME: Adolescent sexual behavior as it relates to other transition behaviors in youth, in Risking the Future: Adolescent Sexuality, Pregnancy, and Childbearing, Vol 2. Edited by Hofferth SL, Hayes CE. Washington, DC, National Academy Press (in press)

Gladis M, Michela JL, Walter HW: Cognitive correlates of high risk AIDS-related behaviors among adolescents: a comparison of theoretical models. Paper presented at the annual meeting of the American Academy of Child and Adolescent Psychiatry, New York, October 1989

Goeddert JJ, Kessler CM, Aledort LM, et al: A prospective study of human immunodeficiency virus type I infection and the development of AIDS in subjects with hemophilia. N Engl J Med 321:1141–1148, 1990

Hayes CE: Risking the Future: Adolescent Sexuality, Pregnancy, and Childbearing. Washington, DC, National Academy Press, 1987

Hayman CR, St. Louis M: HIV Seroprevalence, Job Corps. Paper presented at the NICHD Technical Review and Planning Meeting on Adolescents and HIV Infection, Bethesda, MD, January 1989

Hearst N, Hulley SB: Preventing the heterosexual spread of AIDS: are we giving our patients the best advice? JAMA 259:2428–2432, 1988

Hein K: AIDS in adolescence: exploring the challenge. J Adolesc Health Care 10:10S–35S, 1989

Hunter J: Violence Against Lesbian and Gay Youth: A Report. New York, Hetrick Martin Institute, 1989

Janz NK, Becker MH: The Health Belief Model: a decade later. Health Educ Q 11:1–47, 1984

Kegeles SM, Adler NE, Irwin CE: Sexually active adolescents and condoms: changes over one year in knowledge, attitudes and use. Am J Public Health 78:460–461, 1988

Kelly JA, St. Lawrence JS, Hood HV, et al: Behavioral intervention to reduce AIDS risk activities. J Consult Clin Psychol 57:60–67, 1989

Kinsey AC, Pomeroy WB, Martin CE: Sexual Behavior in the Human Male. Philadelphia, PA, WB Saunders, 1948

Kipke M, Boyer C, Hein K: An evaluation of an AIDS Risk Reduction Education & Skills Training (ARREST) program for adolescents. Paper presented at the 5th International Conference on AIDS, Montreal, Quebec, Canada, June 1989

Koopman C, Rotheram-Borus MJ, Henderson R, et al: Assessment of knowledge and beliefs about AIDS prevention among adolescents. AIDS: Education and Prevention—An Interdisciplinary Journal 2(1):58–70, 1990

Marzuk P, Tierney H, Tardiff K, et al: Increased risk of suicide in persons with AIDS. JAMA 259:1332–1333, 1988

New York City Health Department: AIDS Surveillance Report. New York, AIDS Surveillance Unit, 1990

Orr DP, Wilbrandt ML, Brack CJ, et al: Reported sexual behaviors and self-esteem among young adolescents. Am J Dis Child 143:86–90, 1989

Otis J, Godin G, Lambert J, et al: Cognitive differences between boys and girls relating to the use of condoms, in Abstracts of the 5th International Conference on AIDS. Ottawa, Ontario, Canada, International Research Development Center, 1989, p 715

Owen WF: Medical problems of the homosexual adolescent. J Adolesc Health Care 6:278–285, 1985

Peters SD, Wyatt GE, Finkelhor D: Prevalence, in Sourcebook on Child Sexual Abuse. Edited by Finkelhor D, Araji S, Baron L, et al. Beverly Hills, CA, Sage, 1986, pp 15–59

Quinn TC, Glasser D, Cannon RO, et al: Human immunodeficiency virus infection among patients attending clinics for sexually transmitted diseases. N Engl J Med 318:197–202, 1988

Rabkin J: Workshop on AIDS and suicide. Presented at the National Institute for Mental Health meeting, Ann Arbor, MI, October 1989

Remafedi G: Adolescent homosexuality: psychosocial and medical implications. Pediatrics 79:331–337, 1987

Rhodes F, Wolitski RJ, Arguelles L: Effectiveness of fear appeals in AIDS-education posters: comparison by race/ethnicity, age, and gender in three populations, in Abstracts of the 5th International Conference on AIDS. Ottawa, Ontario, Canada, International Development Research Center, 1989, p 849

Rickert VI, Jay MS, Gottlieb A, et al: Adolescents and AIDS: females' attitudes and behaviors toward condom purchase and use. J Adolesc Health Care 10:313–316, 1989

Rothenberg R: Talking too tough on life's risks? New York Times, February 16, 1990, pp D1, D17

Rotheram-Borus MJ, Koopman C: HIV and adolescents. Journal of Primary Prevention 12:65–82, 1991

Rotheram-Borus MJ, Koopman C, Bradley JS: Barriers to successful AIDS prevention programs with runaway youth, in Troubled Adolescents and HIV Infection: Issues in Prevention and Treatment. Edited by Woodruff JO, Doherty D, Athey JG. Washington, DC, CASSP Technical Assistance Center, 1989a, pp 37–55

Rotheram-Borus MJ, Koopman C, Haignere C, et al: Evaluation of AIDS prevention intervention targeting runaway and gay adolescents (poster). New York, American Academy of Child and Adolescent Psychiatry, October 1989b

Rotheram-Borus MJ, Selfridge C, Koopman C, et al: The relationship of knowledge and attitudes towards AIDS to safe sex practices among runaway and gay adolescents, in Abstracts of the 5th International Conference on AIDS. Ottawa, Ontario, Canada, International Development Research Center, 1989c, p 728

Rotheram-Borus MJ, Rosario M, Koopman C: Minority youths at high risk: gay males and runaways, in Adolescents, Stress and Coping. Edited by Gore S, Colton ME. New York, Aldine Press, 1991, pp 181–200

Sandberg DE, Rotheram-Borus MJ, Bradley J, et al: Methodological issues in assessing AIDS prevention programs. J Adolesc Res 3:413–418, 1988

Seifert-McLean C: University of Maryland, Baltimore, study of HIV seroprevalence in adolescents with sexually transmitted diseases. Paper presented at the NICHD Technical Review and Research Planning Meeting on Adolescents and HIV Infection, Bethesda, MD, January 1989

Shaffer D, Caton C: Runaway and Homeless Youth in New York City. New York, Ittelson Foundation, 1984

Stall RD, Coates TJ, Hoff C: Behavioral risk reduction for HIV infection among gay and bisexual men. Am Psychol 43:878–885, 1988

St. Louis ME, Hayman CR, Miller C, et al: HIV infection in disadvantaged adolescents in the U.S.: findings from the Job Corps Screening Program, in Abstracts of the 5th International Conference on AIDS. Ottawa, Ontario, Canada, International Research Development Center, 1989, p 711

Stricof R, Novick LF, Kennedy J, et al: Seroprevalence at a homeless facility. Paper presented at the American Public Health Association Conference, November 1988

Strunin L, Hingson R: Acquired immunodeficiency syndrome and adolescents: knowledge, beliefs, attitudes and behaviors. Pediatrics 79:825–828, 1987

Trautman P, Shaffer D: Treatment of child and adolescent suicide attempters, in Suicide in the Young. Edited by Sudak H, Ford A, Rushforth N. London, John-Wright–PSG, 1984, pp 307–324

Valdiserri RO, Lyter DW, Leviton LC, et al: AIDS prevention in homosexual and bisexual men: results of a randomized trial evaluating two risk reduction interventions. AIDS 3:21–26, 1989

Zelnick M, Kantner JF: Sexual activity, contraceptive use and pregnancy among metropolitan-area teenagers, 1971–1979. Fam Plann Perspect 12:230–237, 1980

Chapter 5

# Children and Adolescents
# With Hemophilia

Roberta Olson, Ph.D.
Heather Huszti, Ph.D.
Mark Chaffin, Ph.D.

*T*he discovery that persons with hemophilia were at high risk for infection with the human immunodeficiency virus (HIV) has had a profound effect on the entire hemophilia community, including patients, their family members, friends, and the health care workers who provide their medical treatment. Some of these effects are unique to hemophilia, whereas others are perhaps characteristic of all HIV-positive individuals.

Many of the psychological and social issues commonly associated with acquired immunodeficiency syndrome (AIDS) are attributable to idiosyncratic characteristics of the populations in which the disease commonly occurs (e.g., intravenous-drug users, homosexual males) and the life-style characteristics of these populations. Much of the psychosocial research on HIV-related issues is confounded with the issues inherent in being an intravenous-drug abuser or a homosexual male, issues that are often of minimal importance among persons with hemophilia (Mason et al. 1988).

The hemophilia population presents its own idiosyncratic issues, including the fact that HIV infection and AIDS are superimposed on a previously existing chronic illness. The child or adolescent with hemophilia has unique experiences with HIV infection. In other regards, the effects are similar to those of any other child or adolescent with HIV infection, including fear of stigmatization, questions about sexuality, need for prevention information, and death and dying issues. Although it is important to focus on the unique features in each cluster of persons at high risk for HIV infection, it is also important to remain aware of the

areas of common ground. These common themes can be found throughout the chapters in this book.

In this chapter, we discuss both the common and the unique issues
faced by all children and adolescents with hemophilia who are HIV
positive. We include a brief historical overview of hemophilia and AIDS,
discussion of mental health and prevention issues for children and adolescents, and consideration of the decision to inform the child or others of
his status.

## Historical Background

Hemophilia is a genetically transmitted, sex-linked disease that is characterized by a deficiency in blood coagulation factors. Individuals with
hemophilia lack a necessary clotting protein that can result in painful
internal hemorrhaging within large muscle groups and joints. The abnormal gene can produce either a deficiency in coagulation factor VIII
(hemophilia A) or factor IX (hemophilia B). The vast majority of individuals with hemophilia A or B are males. Von Willebrand's disease is a
deficiency in both platelet functioning and factor VIII and can occur in
both men and women.

Treatment of hemophilia A and B involves intravenous infusions of
the missing blood clotting factor. In general, individuals who are defi-
cient in factor VIII (hemophilia A) experience more frequent bleeding
episodes and require more factor-concentrate infusions. In 1984, it was
discovered that persons with hemophilia were also at risk for AIDS
(Centers for Disease Control 1984). Before 1986, the clotting factor was
manufactured through the collection of thousands of individual blood
donations from which the specific factor was removed. Therefore, each
transfusion contained blood clotting factor originating from thousands of
separate donors. A single HIV-positive donor in the pool could infect an
entire batch of clotting factor. The enormity of the problem was demonstrated in a study of one batch of HIV-infected factor VIII concentrate
that was provided to 33 individuals with hemophilia A. Fifteen of the
patients became HIV positive as a result of this batch of infected factor
concentrate. The probability of seroconversion was positively correlated
with the total amount of factor used and the number of transfusions of
infected factor concentrate (Ludlam et al. 1985).

Persons with von Willebrand's disease had a lower risk of becoming
HIV positive than persons with hemophilia A or B. One of the reasons

for this is that the treatment of choice for von Willebrand's disease is cryoprecipitate or fresh frozen plasma that is derived from a single donor. The likelihood of having an HIV-positive donor was much less than for individuals who used factor concentrate. The Bureau of Maternal and Child Health estimates that hemophilia occurs once in every 7,500 live male births. There are presently approximately 20,000 males with hemophilia (13,000 with hemophilia A, 4,000 with von Willebrand's disease, and 3,000 with hemophilia B). In 1987, initial HIV testing of patients seen in hemophilia treatment centers revealed that approximately 92% of tested individuals with severe hemophilia A and 52% of those with hemophilia B were HIV positive (Stehr-Green et al. 1988). Current estimates suggest that 10,000–12,000 persons with hemophilia are HIV positive (National Hemophilia Foundation, personal communication, June 19, 1990). Approximately 50% of persons with hemophilia B are HIV positive, and 70% of those with hemophilia A are HIV positive. For those persons with severe hemophilia A, the percentage rises to approximately 85–90% who are HIV positive. In addition, approximately 15–20% (approximately 1,300 persons) of spouses or sex partners of persons with hemophilia are also HIV positive.

As of April 2, 1990, a total of 1,833 persons with hemophilia were diagnosed with AIDS. Of this total, 175 were below age 13 years. An additional 668 were between ages 13 and 29 years. The risk of HIV infection also runs to the newborn children of HIV-positive persons with hemophilia and their spouses or sex partners. As of April 2, 1990, seven newborns of HIV-positive persons with hemophilia and their sex partners were infected with HIV.

Since 1986, all blood products have been screened for HIV and a heat inactivation process has been employed in manufacturing factor concentrate, virtually eliminating the threat of viral spread through blood products. A recent report from the Centers for Disease Control (1988) notes that since 1986 there have been only six documented seroconversions among patients without any previous exposure to unheated products, and only one of these patients was from the United States. In addition, more purified factor concentrates are now available, and a synthetic factor VIII concentrate is currently undergoing clinical tests. These new products should eliminate the risk of disease transmission through factor concentrate. Tragically, however, an entire cohort of individuals with hemophilia was infected before 1986.

## Hemophilia Treatment Centers

Comprehensive hemophilia treatment centers provide treatment for approximately two-thirds of all individuals with hemophilia. They have been continuously funded by the federal government through Title XI since 1975 (Goldsmith 1986; Levine 1988). The centers provide evaluation, medical management, and psychosocial support for patients and their families. The core treatment team typically consists of a hematologist, a nurse coordinator, and a social worker. Consultation is provided by orthopedic surgeons, dentists, physical therapists, genetic counselors, and psychologists or psychiatrists. More recently, immunologists and infectious disease specialists have also been added to the comprehensive care team to address problems related to HIV infection (Mason et al. 1988).

Persons with hemophilia often have been followed by the same treatment center since childhood, leading to strong patient-staff bonds and an almost familial atmosphere. The core team members grow to know the patients and their families over time and typically establish positive and supportive relationships. Traditionally, individuals with hemophilia have been secretive about their disease due to public misconceptions and biases. Treatment center staff were often the only individuals, outside of the patient's family, who were aware of the patient's disease. Consequently, the patient-staff relationship was often quite private and close-knit. The introduction of HIV infection into the hemophilia population gave impetus to an already-established sense of insularity. Many families and staff continue to remember the experience of the Ray family, whose house was burned by an arsonist in 1986 after they attempted to place their three HIV-positive hemophiliac sons in public school.

Some HIV-positive children have been met with reactions ranging from ambivalence to outright discrimination from the general medical community. The close, protective, and supportive relationship between individuals with hemophilia and treatment center staff is a unique asset (Kelly et al. 1987a, 1987b). As beneficial as this can be, however, it can paradoxically increase the stress experienced by both family and staff. Protectiveness may inadvertently encourage dependency and reliance on the treatment team as the sole source of support. The family may become overly enmeshed with the treatment center, thereby limiting the formation or utilization of indigenous supports. This observation has received empirical support from the finding that hemophilia patients and family members are most likely to use the treatment center as their source of social support and information, while showing minimal desire to become involved with other potential resources (Mason et al. 1989). Reliance on the center can also lead to staff stress, as staff members come to feel increasingly responsible for meeting all psychosocial needs for all their patients. Many treatment center staff have been caught between their wish to protect and insulate and their recognition that outside supports must be developed.

## Outside Consultants

Although the HIV issue has made the treatment center more insular, it has also necessitated the introduction of new professionals and services into the system. It can be difficult for an outside professional to enter into a closed system. Entering consultants should consider two preliminary issues. First, a consultant should be invited into the system by the members of the hemophilia treatment center, with a stated consensus regarding the role for the consultant within the system. It is critical that neither staff nor patients perceive the consultant as someone imposed on them from outside. Second, it is important to realize that patients and family members are often extremely knowledgeable about their medical condition. The consultant should have a good working knowledge of the medical aspects of hemophilia, HIV, and their treatment in order to establish credibility and a shared language.[1]

Once having entered the system, it is important to ascertain team members' philosophies and beliefs. With the advent of HIV, many new and emotional issues have confronted treatment center staff. For example, if the HIV-positive sexual partner of an HIV-positive patient becomes pregnant, should the staff discuss the option of abortion? (See Chapter 1 for further discussion of this issue.) Treatment centers have also struggled with the issue of how to present HIV-prevention information to patients. Should patients be advised against any form of intercourse, even with a condom, because of the possible risk of infection? Should a patient's sexual partners be informed of their risk of HIV

---

[1]Detailed information on hemophilia, its effects on families, and on comprehensive care is available from the National Hemophilia Foundation, 110 Greene Street, New York, NY 10012.

infection? Should staff attempt to trace HIV-positive patients' sexual contacts? Given the potential for any of these questions to generate a heated emotional discourse, it is important to understand staff members' positions before designing an intervention. The consultant may wish to inquire about 1) how HIV-prevention information is dispersed, 2) how aggressively HIV is treated medically, 3) how policies on patient confidentiality are handled, 4) how staff typically inform children and adolescents of their antibody status, and 5) how death and sexuality are discussed.

Consultants should also consider the implications of their formal role in the system, particularly the difference between functioning as a member of the treatment center team as opposed to an outside referral source. In some hemophilia treatment centers, mental health professionals function as formal members of the hemophilia treatment center staff, providing direct services to patients or consulting with team members. In other cases, professionals have no formal role within the hemophilia treatment center and are used as an outside referral source for patients with particular problems.

Each role within the treatment team can have its respective advantages and disadvantages, depending on the patient. Team members may be perceived as credible and trustworthy by patients whose relationships with the treatment center are generally positive. Also, team members have access to more information about the patient and his history and can communicate informally with other members of the team. However, the treatment team psychiatrist or psychologist may be expected to disclose otherwise confidential information to other treatment center staff. This is most often an issue where high-risk sexual behaviors are concerned. Treatment centers are mandated by the federal government to provide HIV-risk-reduction services to seropositive men with hemophilia, and mental health professionals are sometimes called on to document a patient's risk of spreading HIV. Patients and families who feel that they need absolute confidentiality may be more comfortable with an outside professional who is under no obligation to communicate with the treatment center. In addition, patients wishing to establish greater independence from the insularity and enmeshment of the treatment center may prefer an outside referral. In any case, it is important to be aware of which role is being assumed and to make the implications for confidentiality clear to the patient and the treatment center staff before initiating an intervention.

# Mental Health Issues

## Coping With HIV and Hemophilia

Overall, current research suggests that the population with HIV and hemophilia copes comparatively well. In fact, their overall level of distress is often lower than that of either their parents or other family members (Agle et al. 1987; Klein and Nimorwicz 1982). Although generally experiencing some degree of significant distress, the evidence suggests that HIV-positive persons with hemophilia are less distressed than other individuals infected with HIV (Brondolo et al. 1986; Kelly and St. Lawrence 1988). Several factors are thought to explain this finding. As discussed previously, many persons with hemophilia and their family members were already involved with comprehensive care services before becoming infected with HIV and possessed strong pre-existing ties with the medical community. Additionally, seropositive persons with hemophilia may receive more social understanding and less prejudice or stigmatization. Compared with individuals who are homosexual or who abuse intravenous drugs, whose disease is all too often judged to be deserved punishment for moral failures, individuals with hemophilia are usually accorded the status of "innocent victims." Consequently, when young men with hemophilia do disclose their HIV status, it is invariably paired with an exculpatory explanation of its contagion through factor infusions. Finally, persons with hemophilia have become acclimated to chronic illness and are adept at living as normal a life as possible in spite of the constraints imposed by their disease. Many of the same coping mechanisms useful in dealing with hemophilia can be helpful in coping with HIV.

Other carryover coping strategies may be less adaptive. For example, it has been found that although many of these patients are aware that most people with hemophilia have been exposed to HIV, few believe that they will eventually develop AIDS (Brondolo et al. 1986). This invites the possibility that the decreased levels of distress noted earlier may be linked to a tendency to ignore or deny the more frightening aspects of HIV infection. Unfortunately, although some degree of denial may be adaptive for living with a chronic illness such as hemophilia, it is potentially much less adaptive for HIV infection, because the patient needs to adhere to strict prevention precautions and more complicated medical regimens.

Despite their comparatively lower levels of distress, this population experiences many of the same problems and has many of the same needs as other children or adolescents with HIV. These issues, and the implications for psychotherapy with the infected child and family, are discussed at length in Chapter 13.

## Discussing the HIV Diagnosis With Children

Although discussing a life-threatening illness is difficult with any child, psychiatrists and psychologists face a particular dilemma when the child is HIV seropositive or is dying of AIDS. Traditional therapeutic goals with a child and family emphasize honest and open communication. The family might be encouraged to discuss the illness, grieve the pending loss of their child, and reassure the child that he will not be alone, in pain, or forgotten. Where AIDS is concerned, these goals are complicated by the realities of public fear and misinformation. Families risk potential abandonment by extended family or friends, loss of housing, or even loss of employment (Seibert et al. 1990). In addition, children face the possibility of being removed from school and isolated from childhood friends as a result of unrealistic fears concerning contagion. Some parents are well prepared for public discrimination and are willing to go to court to ensure that their child is allowed to continue in school. Others are not. Still others are unwilling to risk telling their child that he has a potentially terminal disease, fearing he will give up hope and hasten his own death. As a result of both societal pressures and parental fears, parents are often reticent to inform their child of his HIV status or the diagnosis of AIDS. Historically, however, hemophilia treatment center staff have been very open about the hemophilia diagnosis and other medical issues. Children are usually told their diagnosis at a young age. They receive instruction on how to self-infuse their own factor concentrate at the first signs of interest. There is a well-developed education package provided by the National Hemophilia Foundation that is used to teach patients and family members about hemophilia and its associated problems (Resnik and Lusher 1988). Although the hemophilia diagnosis is seldom publicly displayed, it is quite openly discussed with the child by staff and family.

HIV infection is another issue. HIV is both less treatable and more socially stigmatized than hemophilia, leading many persons who would readily discuss hemophilia issues to avoid disclosure of HIV status. Parents or staff may feel that the child already has enough to deal with by having hemophilia and fear that he will be overwhelmed if he has to face AIDS as well. Two factors are potentially unique contributors to this reluctance among the parents of children with hemophilia. Some parents are already extremely protective, if not overly protective, of their child. It is fairly well known clinic lore that many of these young men are seldom seen outside the company of their mothers. From earliest childhood, their mothers and fathers have watched vigilantly to see that their son is not physically injured, bumped, bruised, or cut. Enforced abstinence from physical exertion or rough-and-tumble play has often been the rule to avoid a bleed. Some boys come to be seen, both by themselves and their parents, as fragile. This pattern of physical protection, once established, can be extended into the social sphere as well. Consistent with a developed pattern of overprotection, parents may decide to protect their son from knowledge of his condition.

Second, given that hemophilia is a sex-linked hereditary condition, mothers may experience some degree of guilt or feeling of responsibility for their son's disease, and by extension his infection with HIV, making open discussion an even more painful prospect. In cases where parents are reluctant to broach the subject with their son, the mental health professional must weigh the rights of the child to know his diagnosis and medical status along with the parents' right to withhold diagnostic information. Past research and clinical experience indicate that school-age children can, in fact, understand and learn to cope with terminal or potentially life-threatening illnesses (Koocher 1980; Nitschke et al. 1982). Mental health professionals often favor discussing disease status with school-age children. Children are invariably sensitive to their parents' reactions and generally can intuit the gravity of the situation, if not its specifics. The emotional distress occurring when a child realizes he has some sort of serious illness that his family will not discuss is often worse than whatever fears specific knowledge might cause. The mental health professional can assist the parents in understanding that their son is not altogether fragile. It can be useful to remind the parents that their son has negotiated medical crises in the past and emphasize his resources for coping with the knowledge of being HIV positive.

Clinical experience with young children has suggested that most children are less anxious and better able to cope with medications, tests, and hospitalizations if the parents provide an explanation of the child's illness. To a limited extent, and with younger children, this can be accomplished without full disclosure. Parents of younger HIV-positive children have sought a position of compromise in which they simply tell the child he has a virus that is making him sick. The parents are then able to discuss the separate opportunistic illnesses such as mouth ulcers or pneumonia as they occur. This approach allows the parents to be open about the present concrete symptoms without having to directly tell the young child he has contracted the AIDS virus.

Many parents are concerned that informing their child will place an undue burden of secrecy on the child or will eventually lead to public awareness of his HIV status and consequent discrimination. Some parents might be willing to inform their young child if they could do so in isolation, but be unwilling to risk a public "leak." Assuming parents do choose to disclose to the child that he is HIV positive or has AIDS, we still do not know the level of cognitive development required for a child to keep such a diagnosis secret from friends, teachers, or extended family, nor the psychological effects this demand would impose. Keeping the secret may be even more difficult for children whose hemophilia is already public, and who are consequently known to be at high risk. At present, parents and professionals alike must rely on their judgment to determine when and how much to tell.

## School Issues

Given that parents and children are fearful of experiencing the same prejudices as the Rays in Florida and Ryan White in Indiana, it is difficult for mental health professionals to advise the family to be open with the community and school. No compelling reason may exist for the school to know about a child's HIV infection, and parents can easily minimize the risk of disclosure. For example, a child on the standard schedule of zidovudine (AZT), 5 times per 24 hours, can be given a 3 A.M. dose of AZT, thereby eliminating the need for a dose during school hours and the concomitant risk that his diagnosis will be guessed. Considering the link between hemophilia and AIDS, many parents are reluctant to inform the school of the former, fearing that the latter will be assumed. However, there may be compelling reasons for the school to be aware of hemophilia, particularly among younger children who may not be mindful of the necessary limitations on their behavior or capable of managing a self-infusion protocol. Teachers and school nurses may need to know the signs of a bleed and how to respond appropriately. The best role for the mental health professional is to help the family decide who they feel they can trust with the knowledge of their child's hemophilia and/or HIV status and structure the necessary medical safeguards within a confidential framework. Nonetheless, parents and children should be prepared for the eventuality of public disclosure. The mental health professional can assist the family in "rehearsing" an adaptive response and can immunize the child against internalizing the potential social rejection.

Children with hemophilia who are known to be HIV positive encounter difficulties in school for various reasons. Many of the legal issues are similar to those faced by all HIV-infected children and are discussed in Chapter 8. One area where mental health professionals can take an active role is in educating school officials and communities about the low risk of HIV transmission from individuals with hemophilia. HIV-seropositive children need to lead as normal a life as possible, including attending school. The child has a legal right to schooling within the least restrictive environment (see Chapter 8). But a recent survey of school board presidents in Oklahoma indicated that school officials are more likely to recommend homebound instruction for HIV-positive children who are less socially desirable, for example, male adolescents doing poorly in school (Ambuel et al. 1989). Mental health professionals are more likely to be working with low-achieving youngsters and become involved in planning meetings at the schools. The psychiatrist or psychologist is in a strong position to advocate for the psychosocial needs of the HIV-positive child. It may be useful to emphasize to school officials that there is no need to fear that casual contact with HIV-infected individuals will spread the virus.

### Prevention Issues

**Children.** HIV-positive children with hemophilia need to have HIV-prevention information. Even those parents who choose not to discuss their child's antibody status with him can provide a preventive education. The comprehensive hemophilia treatment centers begin educating families about hemophilia from the initial diagnosis. Children can be taught how to properly clean any blood spills from open wounds or injuries and to understand that other people should not touch their blood. Those who have begun to self-administer factor concentrate need to be aware of proper disposal procedures for needles, syringes, intravenous tubing, and factor-concentrate solutions used in self-infusion. The use of proper hygiene with blood spills and self-infusions is important for all children with hemophilia. Even those who are not HIV positive have probably been exposed to the hepatitis B virus and other contaminants through factor-concentrate infusions and can transmit diseases to others. These general precautions also guard against blood-to-blood transmission of HIV.

Prevention of sexual transmission is a more difficult prospect. Ideally, parents and professionals should begin talking with children about sexuality early on, laying the foundation for later discussions of safer sex and HIV prevention. Early discussions teach children that they can openly discuss sex within the family, making it more likely that, as adolescents, they will be able to talk with their parents or other adults. Additionally, parents and/or professionals can start to teach children independent decision-making and problem-solving skills, increasing the likelihood of good decisions about sexual activity and drug use. As adolescence approaches, children can be given specific information and skills pertinent to HIV contagion. Children need information about how to prevent transmission *before* they ever engage in risky behaviors. It is much easier to incorporate prevention strategies into early sexual behaviors than to modify habitually unsafe practices.

**Adolescents.** HIV-positive adolescents with hemophilia represent a high-risk group for spreading the virus to others through unprotected sexual intercourse and drug use (Hein 1989). Adolescents in general are a particularly difficult group to educate about prevention of HIV (Huszti et al. 1989; Melton 1988). This age-group is in the process of moving away from the family, seeking independence, and experimenting with a variety of new behaviors, including sex and drug use. Many adolescents tend to believe that they are invulnerable to personal harm, a perception supported by the fact that they are unlikely to have experienced negative consequences from their risky health behaviors (Elkind 1967; Melton 1987). In addition, peers can subtly or blatantly encourage experimentation with sex and drug use, both of which increase risk of HIV contagion. Chapter 4 discusses the general issues of adolescents and AIDS.

Adolescents with hemophilia experience the same peer pressure, sense of invulnerability, and need to become independent from their families as other adolescents. Beyond this, many feel a need to prove that they are normal in spite of their chronic illness. Having been discouraged from participating in contact sports due to risk of injury, sexual activity can become one vehicle for establishing normality and masculinity.

Sexual activity can also serve as a mode of rebellion against both the limits imposed by their disease(s) and a childhood of parental overprotection and enmeshment. For others, overprotection and enforced abstinence from many normal childhood interactions with peers have delayed social development. Sexual activity may be a way to feel accepted by peers.

As has been seen in other adolescents, education of the hemophiliac population has not resulted in significant behavior change. In a recent study (Overby et al. 1989), all of the HIV-positive adolescents with hemophilia, ages 13–19, demonstrated a high level of knowledge about AIDS. Of the 26 participating in the study, 9 were sexually active. All 9 agreed that using condoms was important to reduce the spread of HIV infection, but only 1 was consistently doing so. Seven reported inconsistent condom use. Of the 6 with steady girlfriends, only 3 had revealed their hemophilia, and only 2 had discussed AIDS issues. Eight of the 26 stated they had abstained from or decreased their sexual activity because of concerns about AIDS. The failure of simple educational programs to effect long-lasting changes in HIV risk behavior is not surprising. The prevention of the spread of HIV involves intervention in complex and essentially private behaviors. Adolescents are just beginning to learn the complexity of romantic and sexual relationships. It may be unrealistic to ask adolescents to introduce the use of condoms and communication about this need into their relationships without offering them training in the skills necessary to accomplish this task. Given the additional emotional, interpersonal, and personality issues involved in the sexual behavior of young men with hemophilia, it is clear that efforts aimed at simply providing HIV contagion information are inadequate. Clearly, prevention efforts need to be much more intensive, skill based, and behavioral.

Previously successful adolescent pregnancy prevention programs have provided both educational and skill-based interventions. These programs have focused on the acquisition of skills necessary to implement the recommended preventive behaviors (Herz et al. 1986; Schnike et al. 1981). Unlike the popular single-session AIDS information programs, effective adolescent sexuality interventions typically require 12–16 sessions. Similarly, AIDS prevention programs need to teach adolescents assertive communication with potential or current sexual partners, appropriate relationship-building skills, and problem-solving skills. Given the necessary skills, adolescents can utilize AIDS-related knowledge and make informed choices. Again, it is much easier to incorporate prevention strategies into early sexual behaviors than it is to modify habitually unsafe practices.

Adolescents' tendency to keep both the hemophilia and HIV diagnoses secret impairs communication, which appears to be crucial to adolescents' use of condoms. A recent study of female adolescents found that condom use was associated with the degree of perceived enjoyment of condoms and the ease of communicating the need to use condoms (Catania et al. 1989). A previous study found a similar relationship between increased communication and the consistent use of contraception (Polit-O'Hara and Kahn 1985).

If the adolescent has an identified sex partner, it can be helpful to include her or him in the educational process. Do not assume that the HIV-positive adolescent will share HIV transmission and safer-sex information with his partner or will be able to present the information accurately (Ragni and Nimorwicz 1989). In addition, the partner may feel uncomfortable discussing or using safer-sex techniques. Inclusion of the sex partner in the education and prevention program increases the couple's ability to effectively communicate and reach mutual decisions about their sexual activity.

Sessions with both members of the couple may be helpful in addressing other underlying issues maintaining participation in high-risk behaviors. A commonly encountered attitude among adolescent sex partners is, "If he's going to die, I want to die too." For these adolescent partners, dying is viewed as the ultimate romantic gesture, a "Romeo and Juliet" syndrome. Believing in their personal invulnerability, the finality of death can be denied. For other HIV-infected adolescents, there is a strong desire to have a child before they die, which leads them to participate in unprotected sexual intercourse. Identifying and addressing the motivations of each partner are important for ensuring the effectiveness of any intervention.

**Celibacy and prevention.**   Some HIV-positive adolescents with hemophilia have made a decision to abstain from all sexual activity for fear of spreading the virus. These adolescents still need to receive prevention information, because decisions regarding sexual behavior are often made impulsively. For some adolescents, the decision to avoid sexual activity may be a symptom of underlying depression, either reactive or primary. Reactive depressions may be caused, in part, by feelings of anticipatory loss or internalization of the AIDS stigma.

For some adolescents, the decision to withdraw may be more complex. As children, they were often overly protected by their parents. As adolescents, they may have not experienced normal interactions with their peers, participated in extracurricular activities, or developed age-appropriate interests or social skills. These youngsters may be rejected by peers because of their immaturity and enmeshment with parents. Consequently, they may decide to withdraw from social relationships, ostensibly in response to HIV status, but more saliently as a welcome relief from further social anxiety and rejection. Training in appropriate social and relationship skills, as well as education about the transmission of HIV, may facilitate peer acceptance and increase self-esteem.

## Summary

Unlike other high-risk populations, HIV-positive children and adolescents with hemophilia represent a socioeconomic and cultural cross-section of America. Uniquely, however, these children have previously had to cope with chronic illness, albeit one that they could expect to survive. With the advent of HIV infection in this population, they have been burdened with an additional chronic illness, one that is both life threatening and has severe social consequences. The mental health consultant who works with this population is faced with a variety of issues. Families and medical staffs have to decide whether to inform children of their diagnosis, when and how much to tell them about HIV infection, and how to approach the issue of sexual contagion. Children and adolescents have to learn how to live with the uncertain course of the disease. Patients, family members, and medical staff also have to face the personal devastation the disease has brought to their lives. Certainly no one working with HIV-positive persons with hemophilia will have any definitive answers about these issues. The task is more one of helping patients, family members, and medical staff delineate the issues and begin to make personal decisions about how best to address them.

## References

Agle D, Gluck H, Pierce GF: The risk of AIDS: psychologic impact on the hemophilic population. Gen Hosp Psychiatry 9:11–17, 1987

Ambuel B, Mullins LL, Johnson J, et al: AIDS education of educators: a model for needs assessment and intervention. Paper presented at the 2nd Florida Conference on Child Health, Gainesville, FL, April 1989

Brondolo E, Clemow L, Saidi P: Assessment of psychosocial needs concerning AIDS in hemophiliacs, their relatives, and staff. Paper presented at the 38th annual meeting of the National Hemophilia Foundation, Washington, DC, September 1986

Catania JA, Dolcini MM, Coates TJ, et al: Predictors of condom use and multiple partnered sex among sexually active adolescent women: implications for AIDS-related health interventions. Journal of Sex Research 26:514–524, 1989

Centers for Disease Control: Update: acquired immunodeficiency syndrome (AIDS) in persons with hemophilia. MMWR 33:589, 1984

Centers for Disease Control: Safety of therapeutic products used for hemophilia patients. MMWR 37:441–444, 1988

Elkind D: Egocentrism in adolescence. Child Dev 38:1025–1034, 1967

Goldsmith M: Hemophilia, beaten on one front, is beset on others (editorial). JAMA 256:3200, 1986

Hein K: AIDS in adolescence. J Adolesc Health Care 10(3S):10S–35S, 1989

Herz EJ, Reis JS, Barbera-Stein L: Family life education for young teens: an assessment of three interventions. Health Educ Q 13:201–221, 1986

Huszti HC, Clopton JR, Mason PJ: Acquired immunodeficiency syndrome educational program: effects on adolescents' knowledge and attitudes. Pediatrics 84:986–994, 1989

Kelly JA, St. Lawrence JS: AIDS prevention and treatment: psychology's role in the health crisis. Clin Psychol Rev 8:255–284, 1988

Kelly JA, St. Lawrence JS, Smith S, et al: Stigmatization of AIDS patients by physicians. Am J Public Health 77:789–791, 1987a

Kelly JA, St. Lawrence JS, Smith S, et al: Medical students' attitudes toward AIDS and homosexual patients. Journal of Medical Education 62:549–556, 1987b

Klein RH, Nimorwicz P: The relationship between psychological distress and knowledge of disease among hemophilia patients and their families: a pilot study. J Psychosom Res 26:387–391, 1982

Koocher GP: Initial consultations with the pediatric cancer patient, in Psychological Aspects of Childhood Cancer. Edited by Kellerman J. Springfield, IL, Charles C Thomas, 1980, pp 232–237

Levine PH (spokesperson): Hemophilia treatment and research (statement by the National Hemophilia Foundation). Testimony submitted to United States House of Representatives Subcommittee on Labor, HHS Appropriations, May 1988

Ludlam CA, Tucker J, Steel CM, et al: Human T-lymphotropic virus type III (HTLV-III) infection in seronegative hemophiliacs after transfusion of factor VIII. Lancet 2:233–236, 1985

Mason PJ, Olson RA, Parish KL: AIDS, hemophilia, and prevention efforts within a comprehensive care program. Am Psychol 43:971–976, 1988

Mason PJ, Olson RA, Myers J, et al: AIDS and hemophilia: implications for interventions with families. J Pediatr Psychol 14:341–355, 1989

Melton GB: Prevention of HIV infection among adolescents. Testimony presented before the United States House of Representatives Select Committee on Children, Youth, and Families, Washington, DC, 1987

Melton GB: Adolescents and the prevention of AIDS. Professional Psychology 19:403–408, 1988

Nitschke R, Humphrey GB, Sexauer CL, et al: Therapeutic choices made by patients with end-stage cancer. J Pediatr 101:471–476, 1982

Overby KJ, Lo B, Litt IF: Knowledge and concerns about acquired immunodeficiency syndrome and their relationship to behaviors among adolescents with hemophilia. Pediatrics 83:204–210, 1989

Polit-O'Hara D, Kahn J: Communication and contraceptive practices in adolescent couples. Adolescence 20:33–43, 1985

Ragni MV, Nimorwicz P: Human immunodeficiency virus transmission and hemophilia. Arch Intern Med 149:1379–1380, 1989

Resnik SG, Lusher J: Education as an Integral Component of Care at Hemophilia Treatment Centers. New York, National Hemophilia Foundation, 1988

Schnike SP, Blythe BJ, Gilchrist LD: Cognitive-behavioral prevention of adolescent pregnancy. Journal of Counseling Psychology 28:451–454, 1981

Seibert JM, Garcia A, Kaplan M, et al: Three model pediatric AIDS programs: meeting the needs of children, families, and communities, in Children, Adolescents, and AIDS. Edited by Seibert JM, Olson RA. Lincoln, University of Nebraska Press, 1990

Stehr-Green JK, Holman RC, Jason JM, et al: Hemophilia-associated AIDS in the United States, 1981 to September 1987. Am J Public Health 78:439–442, 1988

# Specific Issues for HIV-Infected Children

## Chapter 6

# Neurologic Aspects

Anita L. Belman, M.D.
Dennis W. Dickson, M.D.

*C*entral nervous system (CNS) involvement and CNS disease related to human immunodeficiency virus type 1 (HIV-1) frequently complicate the course of symptomatic HIV-1 infection and acquired immunodeficiency syndrome (AIDS) in infants and children (Belman et al. 1988; Epstein et al. 1988a). Indeed, it has been estimated that within the next several years, HIV-1–related CNS disease may become one of the leading infectious causes of mental deficiency and developmental disabilities in infants and children in some geographical regions of the United States (Diamond 1989).

HIV-1 belongs to the lentivirus subfamily of nononcogenic retroviruses. These "slow viruses" cause persistent infection and chronic disease. Nervous system involvement has a slow and progressive course (Johnson et al. 1988). Because HIV-1 is both lymphotropic and neurotropic, it causes a wide spectrum of disease in infants and children (Falloon et al. 1989; Rubinstein 1986). The most severe form of the disease results in AIDS.

The CNS in HIV-1–infected infants and children may be affected by 1) pathologic processes related to primary HIV-1 CNS infection—HIV-1 itself—or 2) pathologic processes related to immunodeficiency—secondary complications that may develop in immunosuppressed patients, including CNS lymphoma, CNS infections caused by pathogens other than HIV-1, and cerebrovascular complications.

The CNS in HIV-1–infected children may also be affected by metabolic complications related to HIV-1 systemic disease. It is important to keep in mind that as new antiretroviral and immunomodulating therapies for HIV-1 become available and as new therapies for HIV-1–associated illnesses are introduced, the possibility exists that CNS complications may also develop from metabolic or toxic effects of these agents.

In addition, the developing CNS of HIV-1–infected infants may be adversely affected by maternal conditions, for example, poor or no prenatal care, inadequate maternal nutrition, or maternal illness(es) during pregnancy. Moreover, the developing nervous system may be adversely affected by in utero exposure to drugs (e.g., heroin, cocaine, crack, alcohol, methadone). In the perinatal period, the low-birth-weight or prematurely born infant is also at risk for developing complications that affect the immature nervous system, such as hypoxic-ischemic encephalopathy, periventricular leukomalacia, and intraventricular and intraparenchymal hemorrhage.

## CNS Complications Associated With Immunodeficiency of HIV-1 Infection

CNS lymphoma, strokes, and CNS infections caused by organisms other than HIV-1 have been well described in children with HIV-1 infection. In our longitudinal study, approximately 18% of patients developed one or more of these CNS complications (Belman et al. 1988; Park et al. 1990). Most of these children also had, or subsequently developed, coexisting encephalopathy related to HIV-1 (Belman et al. 1988).

### Neoplasm

Primary CNS lymphoma and systemic lymphoma metastatic to the CNS are now well-recognized neurological complications in children with HIV-1 infection (Belman et al. 1988, 1990; Dickson et al. 1989, 1990; Epstein et al. 1988b). Focal neurologic deficits, seizures, and changes in mental status are the most common presenting signs. In some children, neurologic deterioration is rapid and fulminant. These signs usually can be distinguished from the more insidious neurologic deterioration characteristic of HIV-1–related encephalopathy discussed later in this chapter (Belman 1990b; Belman et al. 1988).

Neuroimaging studies in children with lymphoma, as in those in adults, may reveal 1) mass lesion(s), with or without surrounding edema, that may or may not enhance with contrast material, 2) diffuse lesions that may or may not be contrast enhancing, or 3) contrast-enhancing periventricular lesions. Both solitary and multiple lesions have been reported.

## Cerebrovascular Complications

Strokes have also been described in children with symptomatic HIV-1 infection (Belman et al. 1988; Frank et al. 1989; Kure et al. 1989; Park et al. 1990). The new onset of focal neurologic deficits, most commonly hemiparesis, at times associated with seizures, is the most common presentation (Park et al. 1990). Neuroradiologic studies reveal findings that are consistent with 1) bland infarction, 2) hemorrhagic infarction, or 3) intracranial hemorrhage.

Nonhemorrhagic infarctions may be associated with 1) meningeal infections, 2) intrinsic disease of cerebral blood vessels, or 3) cardiomyopathy (Dickson et al. 1989, 1990; Frank et al. 1989; Kure et al. 1989; Park et al. 1990).

Intracerebral hemorrhage is usually associated with immune-mediated thrombocytopenia. The severity and location of hemorrhage dictate clinical presentation. Seizures, changes in mental status, focal neurologic deficits, and/or signs of increased intracranial pressure have been described. Strokes may be catastrophic and fatal, although clinically silent events have also been reported (Belman et al. 1988; Park et al. 1990).

## CNS Infections

Opportunistic infections of the CNS are not as common in HIV-1–infected infants and children as they are in HIV-1–infected adults (Belman et al. 1988; Dickson et al. 1989; Sharer et al. 1986). However, serious bacterial infections, including meningitis, do occur in children with AIDS (Bernstein et al. 1985; Rubinstein 1986). Neurologic sequelae are variable and may include varying degrees of sensorineural hearing loss and cognitive and motor impairment of varying severity (Belman 1990; Belman et al. 1988).

*Candida albicans* is the most common fungal infection reported; both meningitis and microabscess have been described. Cytomegalovirus (CMV) encephalitis is the most common viral CNS infection documented (Belman et al. 1985, 1988; Epstein et al. 1988a). The role of coinfection (e.g., herpesvirus and HIV-1) and/or transactivation remains to be elucidated.

# HIV-1–Related CNS Disease

## Background

As children with AIDS were followed longitudinally, it became evident that in the majority of patients the stereotypic CNS impairment (described below) was not due to the secondary complications of immunodeficiency or the metabolic complications of systemic disease. It also seemed that by the time HIV-1 infection had advanced to severe symptomatic stages, cognitive, behavioral, and motor deficits of varying severity, duration, and progression were frequent findings. During the same period, evidence accumulated from various laboratory and neuropathologic studies indicated that the CNS was directly infected by HIV-1 (Epstein et al. 1985; Gabuzda et al. 1986; Goudsmit et al. 1986; Ho et al. 1985; Levy et al. 1985; Pumarola-Sune et al. 1987; Resnick et al. 1985; Shaw et al. 1985; Wiley et al. 1986, 1990). This suggested that HIV-1 was the causative agent for AIDS dementia complex (adults) and AIDS/HIV-1 encephalopathy (children) (Belman et al. 1985, 1988; Epstein et al. 1985, 1987; Navia et al. 1986).

## Incidence

The incidence and prevalence of HIV-1–related CNS disease in children infected with HIV-1 are not known. Current estimates have been derived from dissimilar cohorts: 1) studies of children with advanced systemic HIV-1 disease (AIDS) as defined by the 1985 criteria of the Centers for Disease Control (CDC), and 2) prospective studies of infants and children with asymptomatic, less symptomatic, and symptomatic HIV-1 disease (1987 CDC criteria). A 50–63% prevalence of HIV-1 encephalopathy is estimated from the first cohorts (Belman et al. 1988; Epstein et al. 1988a). A significantly lower prevalence of progressive neurological disease (9–31%) is estimated from the second cohort (European Collaborative Study 1990; Blanche et al. 1990). However, the mean age of children in this latter group was somewhat younger than the former, and many children's HIV-1 disease had not yet progressed to severe symptomatic stages (AIDS or AIDS-related complex [ARC]). Although it has been the impression of clinicians that CNS involvement is more frequent in children with advanced systemic HIV-1 disease, confirmation of this observation must await completion of prospective studies.

The incidence of "static" encephalopathy (see below) is also not known. A 25% prevalence has been reported (Belman et al. 1988; Epstein et al. 1988a; Hittelman et al. 1989).

## Neurologic Findings and Course of HIV-1–Related CNS Disease

The most frequent neurologic findings in HIV-1–infected children include cognitive impairment, developmental delays, acquired microcephaly, and bilateral corticospinal tract signs (Belman et al. 1985, 1988; Epstein et al. 1986). Movement disorders and signs of cerebellar dysfunction occur, but less frequently (Belman et al. 1988).

Two forms of encephalopathy were initially described and broadly classified as *progressive* or *static* (Belman et al. 1985, 1988; Epstein et al. 1985, 1986; Ultmann et al. 1985, 1987). Our continued clinical observations suggested that the progressive course could be further divided into subtypes based again on progression and severity of encephalopathic findings (Figure 6–1). These subtypes were termed 1) subacute progressive, 2) plateau, 3) plateau followed by further deterioration, and 4) plateau followed by improvement (Belman et al. 1988, 1990).

It was also noted that in some children there was a marked discrepancy between progression and severity of motor dysfunction compared with more stable, albeit impaired, cognitive, language, and socially adaptive abilities (Belman 1990; Belman et al. 1985).

### HIV-1 Encephalomyelopathy

In infants and young children, CNS involvement may first be manifested by deterioration of play and loss of previously acquired language and socially adaptive skills (Figure 6–1, *A*). Progressive motor dysfunction is common (Belman et al. 1985, 1988). The infant may lose previously acquired motor skills, become spastic, or show marked delays in acquisition of new motor skills (Belman 1990; Belman et al. 1985, 1988, 1990; Epstein et al. 1985, 1986). The toddler or young child may develop a change in gait, may begin to toe walk (a sign of increased extensor tone), or may even refuse to walk at all (Belman 1990). These progressive corticospinal tract signs may result in incapacitating spastic quadriparesis with pseudobulbar signs. Rigidity, dystonic posturing, and/or extrapyramidal tremor have also been described. Some children develop

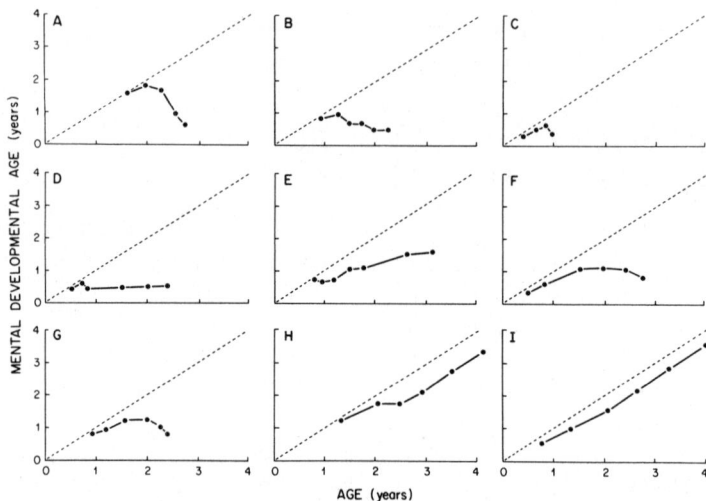

**Figure 6–1.** "Encephalopathic" courses of nine patients. *Dashed line* represents "normal" mental development. *Dotted line* represents patient's mental developmental age. From Belman AL: AIDS and pediatric neurology. Neurol Clin 8:571–603, 1990. Reprinted with permission.

cerebellar signs. A characteristic facial appearance develops in some children. There is a paucity of spontaneous facial expression although there is no facial weakness as evidenced by full movement when crying (Belman 1990). As HIV-1 CNS disease advances, eventually children become apathic, lose interest in their environment, and have decreased gestures and vocalizations. The child at end stage is mute, dull-eyed, and quadriparetic.

In other children, neurologic deterioration is episodic (intermittent). The child has periods of deterioration that are interrupted by variable periods of relative neurologic stability (Figure 6–1, *B*).

In some children, neurologic deterioration occurs fairly rapidly over a period of weeks and may result in severe neurologic deficits (Belman 1990; Belman et al. 1988) (Figure 6–1, *C* and *D*).

However, in most children, neurologic deterioration is more indolent. CNS dysfunction becomes evident only as the rate of mental development declines. As can be seen from Figure 6–1, *E* and *F,* over time the infant or young child gains few or no further cognitive skills. This course was originally described as *plateau.* New milestones are either not acquired, or the rate of acquisition of new milestones deviates not only from the norm, but also from the child's previous rate of early developmental progress (Belman et al. 1988). IQ scores, or in the younger child the Mental Developmental Index of the Bayley Scales of Infant Development (Bayley 1969), decline. However, the mental developmental age of the child may remain the same for months and then gradually increase (Belman et al. 1989, 1990). Motor involvement is common, but the progression and severity vary.

Poor brain growth can be documented by serial head-circumference measurements. When plotted on standardized growth charts (such as in Nellhaus 1968), there is downward deviation and crossing of percentile curves (Belman et al. 1985, 1988).

Unfortunately, with disease progression, many of these patients (plateau) will also have further neurologic deterioration (further loss of language, socially adaptive skills, and/or motor skills) (Figure 6–1, *F* and *G*) (Belman et al. 1988).

Interestingly, a minority of children, who previously had declining rates of development or developmental arrest, showed improvement (Belman et al. 1988) (Figure 6–1, *H*). Follow-up examinations in these children documented acquisition of additional cognitive and developmental skills. Such children functioned in the moderate, mild, or borderline range of mental retardation (IQ of 50–79). Long tract signs, when present, remained stable during follow-up. Thus, this pattern resembled static encephalopathy (Figure 6–1, *I*); however, as in plateau, it is unclear if the rate of CNS maturation was exceeding the slower rate of deterioration or if the disease was quiescent at this point.

Loss of interest in school performance, attention deficits or worsening of attention deficits, psychomotor slowing, social withdrawal, increased emotional lability, and, in some children, attention deficits, hyperactivity, and conduct disorders have been described as early manifestations of HIV-1–related CNS disease in older children (Belman 1990; Belman et al. 1986; Loveland and Stehbens 1990). Long tract signs of varying progression and severity are common. Movement disorders and/or signs of cerebellar involvement may also occur (Belman et al. 1986, 1988). At end stage, there is apathy, cognitive impairment, reduced spontaneous vocalization, and motor dysfunction.

## "Static" Encephalopathy

Early in the AIDS epidemic, it was noted that many children with AIDS or ARC had histories of delays in acquisition of language and motor milestones with subsequent cognitive and motor impairment of varying severity (Belman et al. 1985, 1988; Ultmann et al. 1985) (Figure 6–1, *I*). Additional studies have confirmed this observation (Diamond 1989; Epstein et al. 1986; Hittleman et al. 1989; Ultmann et al. 1987). Most children function in the low-normal, borderline, or mild range of mental retardation. Of these, most also have various degrees of motor involvement. Nonprogressive cognitive and motor impairment have been documented on serial neurologic and psychometric assessments (Belman et al. 1988; Diamond 1990; Ultmann et al. 1987). Children continued to acquire additional developmental skills at a fairly steady rate during the 4-year follow-up. IQ scores remained stable, as did motor deficits. Many children also had signs of attention deficits with or without hyperactivity. Head-circumference measurements in the majority of these patients were below the 50th percentile (range 2–25). However, serial measurements confirmed continued and stable brain growth (Belman et al. 1988).

We initially described this subset of children as having a "static" course. It must be kept in mind that the children were not followed prospectively from birth. Thus, it is possible that some children may have had an undocumented encephalopathy (related or not related to HIV-1 CNS infection) in infancy or early childhood (Belman 1990). Many of the children also had in utero exposure to drugs. Moreover, some children described as having static encephalopathy were said to have been born prematurely, and therefore, presumably, a subset of these children may have had CNS complications associated with prematurity. These confounding issues have made analysis difficult, and it is unclear what role they play in this impairment (Belman et al. 1988).

## Neuroimaging Findings

Computed tomography (CT) of the head in children with HIV-1–related CNS disease shows variable degrees of cerebral atrophy and white matter abnormalities (low density) (Belman et al. 1985, 1988; Epstein et al. 1985). Some infants and children also have bilateral symmetrical calcification of the basal ganglia and, less frequently, calcification of the frontal white matter (Belman et al. 1986). Serial studies in children who lost milestones in general show progressive atrophy and white matter abnormalities (Belman 1990; Belman et al. 1988, 1990) (Figure 6–2). Some children have progressive calcification of the basal ganglia (Belman et al. 1986). Magnetic resonance imaging (MRI) reveals atrophy and increased abnormal signal intensity in the white matter on T2 weighted images (Belman 1990; Belman et al. 1986). Abnormal signal may also be noted in the deep gray structures. MRI may show abnormalities in the white matter and deep gray structures that are not visualized on CT or that, when present on CT, may appear more extensive on MRI (Belman 1990).

In some children with plateau, CT may be normal or may show atrophy (Belman 1990; Wiley et al. 1990). White matter changes, when present, are usually mild. Serial studies may not show progressive changes (Wiley et al. 1990). MRI studies in children with declining developmental progress or developmental arrest may show abnormal high signal in the basal ganglia and the white matter (Belman et al. 1990).

Children with static encephalopathy usually have normal CT studies or CT showing mild atrophy. Serial studies have not documented progressive changes. However, MRI studies have been abnormal in some children (Belman 1990).

## Neuropathology

The pathological findings of CNS involvement in symptomatic HIV infection have been described in adults (Navia et al. 1986; Petito et al. 1985) and children (Dickson et al. 1989; Sharer et al. 1986). The best documented effect of HIV-1 infection of the CNS is a productive infection of microglia, resulting in the formation of multinucleated giant cells. There is also frequent damage to myelin, best recognized in the form of diffuse myelin pallor in the cerebral white matter, and in adults by vacuolar degeneration in the spinal cord. There are, however, several ways in which adults and children differ.

First, HIV-1 infection in adults occurs in mature individuals, with fully developed and completely myelinated nervous systems. The immune system is also mature and the intrinsic microglia, CNS elements of the mononuclear phagocyte system, are highly ramified cells in a quiescent or resting state. Second, adults have had a variety of life experiences that have exposed them to infectious agents that are held in check by an intact host response. Examples of these agents are CMV, toxoplasma, and papovavirus.

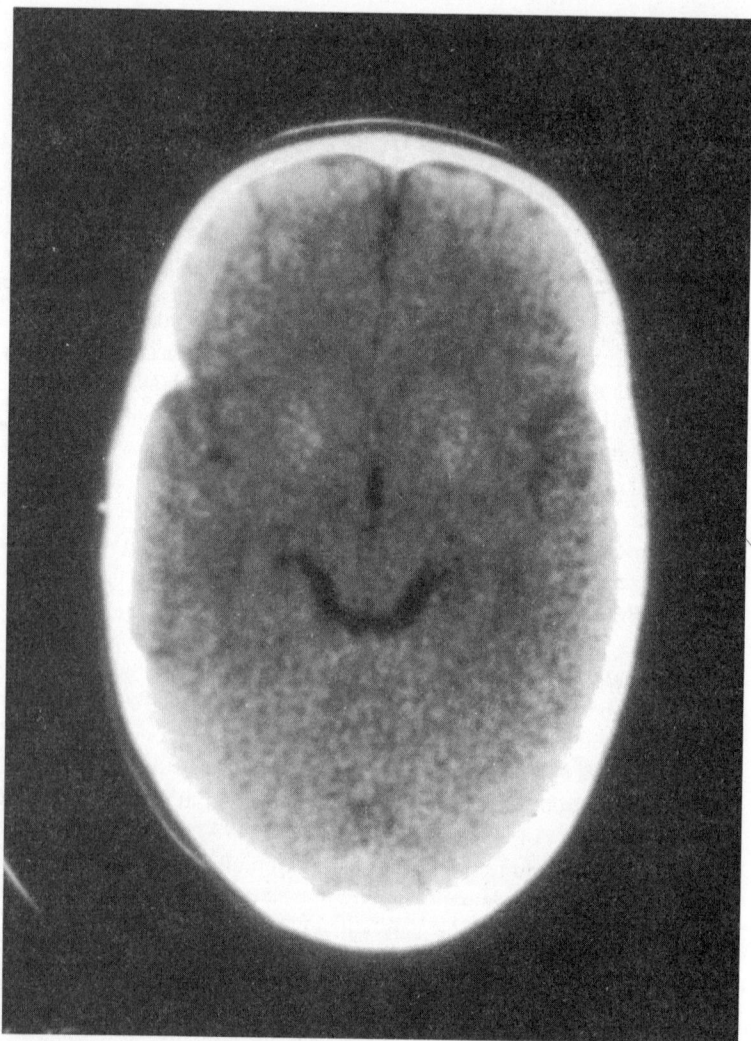

**Figure 6–2.** *Left:* Computed tomography (CT) scan of child at age 14 months with HIV-1 encephalopathy shows faint calcification of the basal ganglia. Examination was remarkable for an alert responsive child who was no longer able to pull to stand, cruise, or walk. Lower-extremity muscle tone was increased and deep tendon reflexes were hyperactive with bilateral ankle clonus.

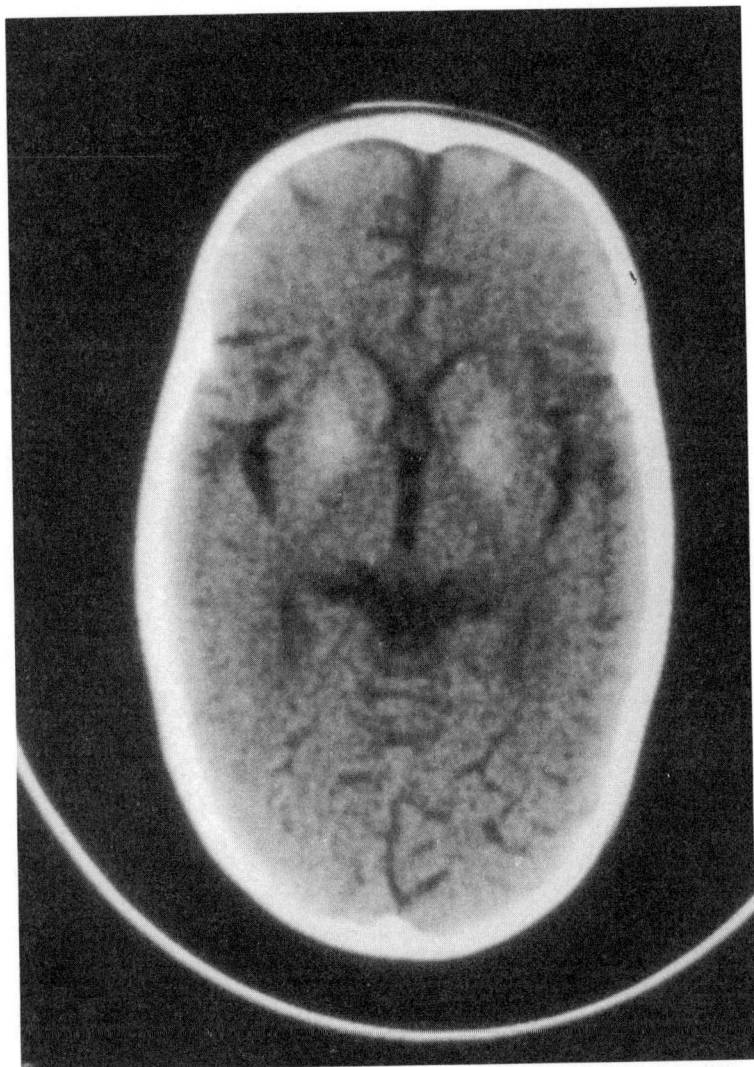

**Figure 6–2.** *Right:* Follow-up CT of same child at age 22 months (8 months later) shows mild cerebral atrophy and progressive calcification of the basal ganglia. Neurologic examination at this time revealed an alert but irritable child with acquired microcephaly, severe language delay, and spastic quadriparesis.

On the other hand, HIV-1 infection in children occurs in an immature and developing organism. Most evidence suggests that HIV-1 infection in children is acquired either transplacentally or during labor and delivery. At these times, the nervous system is in a state of cellular proliferation, migration, and differentiation. These events do not occur uniformly throughout the nervous system. Some neurons are still actively dividing and migrating in the newborn, whereas others are fully mature at birth. Cerebellar granular neurons continue migration to their final location well into the second year of life. In addition, myelination is incomplete in the infant or young child. The corticospinal tract, for example, is incompletely myelinated until nearly age 2 years. Other cortical-association fiber systems do not completely myelinate until young adulthood.

Infants and young children also have not been exposed to the variety of infectious agents to which most adults have been exposed. CMV and toxoplasma infections in the pediatric population are primary infections, rather than reactivation infections typical of adults. Although CMV and toxoplasmosis are common CNS complications in adults, CMV and toxoplasma (primary) infections have not been frequently described in pediatric AIDS.

The immune system of the fetus or neonate is immature during the initial exposure to HIV-1. Less is known about the status of the mononuclear phagocytic cell population in the developing human nervous system, but evidence suggests that microglia are present in the fetus by at least 13 weeks and probably as early as 6 weeks of gestational age. Microglial maturation, however, is probably incomplete in the neonate. The neonate is also relatively immunodeficient with respect to humoral immunity, having low levels of complement factors and immunoglobulins, which are largely derived from maternal antibodies, so that children are more apt to be infected by bacterial agents (e.g., bacterial meningitis) than are adults.

It has proved difficult to document productive HIV-1 infection in microglia in children compared with adults, using the same techniques and reagents and tissue processed in a similar manner (Kure et al. 1990). Vacuolar degeneration is also far less common in children and in one report was only detected in an older child with mature myelin (Dickson et al. 1989). This suggested that some of the damaging effects of HIV infection on myelin may to some extent be dependent on the maturity of myelin.

In further support of this concept, children often show myelin pathology that is selective for fiber tracts that are last to myelinate. One of the most characteristic findings in the nervous system in pediatric AIDS is symmetrical corticospinal tract degeneration in the spinal cord (Dickson et al. 1989). Although somewhat similar findings have been described in adults with AIDS, they are less common. These results have suggested that HIV-1 infection may be either directly or indirectly injurious to newly formed myelin or myelinating glia.

The time course of the disease process is clearly different in adults and children. Although inflammatory disease of the CNS (so-called AIDS subacute encephalitis) characterized by lymphohistiocytic infiltrates, especially around blood vessels in the white matter and the deep gray matter and multinucleated giant cells, has been described in adults and children, the extent of AIDS encephalitis in children has been reported to be directly related to the child's age. Older children more often had active infiltrates, whereas younger children and infants usually had a paucity of such changes, even when they had clinically apparent disease. Although HIV-1 infection in adults appears to be associated with a prolonged incubation period and a protracted clinical course lasting for several years, in some children with vertically transmitted HIV-1 the incubation period is remarkably short. Although limited in extent, we have seen inflammatory infiltrates with multinucleated giant cells in infants as young as age 5 months. This suggests that the fetal and infant brain may be innately more susceptible to a more rapid disease process.

A common finding in the CNS of children with symptomatic HIV-1 infection is acquired microcephaly and progressive mineralization in the basal ganglia and frontal white matter. The mechanism of this process is unclear, but light and electron microscopic findings suggest that in most cases the mineralization is present in the walls of small and medium-size blood vessels. This dystrophic calcification suggests that blood vessels may be damaged in HIV-1 infection. Whether this is due to direct viral infection or indirect effects has not been determined with certainty. Attempts to localize HIV-1 antigens to endothelial cells have been met with limited success; the major cell type expressing viral antigens has been localized to blood vessels in at least one case of CNS aneurysmal arteriopathy in pediatric AIDS (Kure et al. 1989).

It is apparent that HIV-1 infection in infants and children is complicated by numerous developmental parameters. The developmental stage of the nervous system and the immune system during which the virus is initially present can be expected to interact in a complex way with variables related to HIV-1, including whether it is a neurotropic strain of HIV.

## Summary

It is now well recognized that HIV-1–related CNS disease may complicate the course of symptomatic HIV-1 infection and AIDS in infants and children. Evidence exists indicating that this stereotypic CNS impairment is related to HIV-1 brain infection, and it appears that the CNS may be infected early in the course of disease. However, it is also well recognized that much remains to be learned about the effects of this retrovirus on the CNS. Moreover, the effects of HIV-1 on the developing CNS and the developing immune system and on the innumerable, dynamic, and complex interactions between these two developing systems must be considered.

The relationship between CNS viral invasion, latency, immune competence, and the subsequent neurologic course remains uncertain. Indeed, the explanation for the varied encephalopathic courses we described, disease progression, and the different pathologic lesions described above are currently unknown. It is most probable that the different pathogenetic mechanisms reflect different clinical expressions of CNS disease (Belman 1990). As reviewed recently by Johnson and colleagues (1988), both direct and indirect effects of HIV-1 have been proposed. These include 1) possible direct effects of HIV-1 infection on neural cells (cytopathic or altering cell function), 2) effects of viral proteins (possibly blocking neuroreceptors or blocking neurotropic factors), 3) effects of macrophages and monocytes, including the effects of cytokines and chemotactic factors and the possible effects of these substances on the function of neurons and glia, 4) effects on endothelial cells possibly resulting in alterations of the blood-brain barrier, 5) activation of other infectious agents, and 6) autoimmunity. Viral strain differences and host-related factors, including coinfection with other pathogens, are probably also involved.

Continuing research efforts are focusing on the timing and route of HIV-1 CNS invasion. Prospective studies are also in progress looking further at the natural history of HIV-1 CNS disease to determine the earliest neurological, neuroimaging, and neurophysiologic manifestations of HIV-1–related CNS disease in infancy and early childhood; to correlate the encephalopathic courses with immunologic and virologic status; and to identify prognostic correlates and surrogate markers. Host, environmental, and viral factors related to disease progression are also under investigation. These studies are critical not only for the design of antiviral and immunomodulating therapeutic protocols but are required to monitor drug efficacy of existing and future therapeutic regimens (Belman 1990).

In summary, the manifestations of HIV-1–related CNS disease are complex and challenging to the clinicians who evaluate and care for these children.

# References

Bayley N: Bayley Scales of Infant Development. San Antonio, TX, Psychological Corporation, 1969

Belman AL: AIDS and pediatric neurology. Neurol Clin 8:571–603, 1990

Belman AL, Ultmann MH, Horoupian D, et al: Neurologic complications in infants and children with acquired immune deficiency syndrome. Ann Neurol 18:560–566, 1985

Belman AL, Lantos G, Horoupian D, et al: AIDS: calcification of the basal ganglia in infants and children. Neurology 36:1192–1199, 1986

Belman AL, Diamond G, Dickson D, et al: Pediatric AIDS: neurologic syndromes. Am J Dis Child 142:29–35, 1988

Belman AL, Diamond G, Park Y, et al: Perinatal HIV infection: a prospective longitudinal study of the initial CNS signs. Neurology 39 (suppl):278–279, 1989

Belman AL, Calvelli T, Nozyce M, et al: Neurologic and immunologic correlates in infants with vertically transmitted HIV infection. Neurology 40 (suppl 1):409, 1990

Bernstein LJ, Krieger BZ, Novick BE, et al: Bacterial infections—the acquired immunodeficiency syndrome in children. Pediatr Infect Dis 4:472–475, 1985

Blanche S, Tardieu M, Duliege A, et al: Longitudinal study of 94 symptomatic infants with perinatally acquired human immunodeficiency infection: evidence for a bimodal expression of clinical and biologic symptoms. Am J Dis Child 144:1210–1215, 1990

Diamond G: Developmental problems in children with HIV infection. Ment Retard 27:213–217, 1989

Diamond GW, Gurdin P, Wiznia AA, et al: Effects of congenital HIV infection on neurodevelopmental status of babies in foster care. Dev Med Child Neurol 32:999–1005, 1990

Dickson DW, Belman AL, Park YD, et al: Central nervous system pathology in pediatric AIDS: an autopsy study. APMIS Suppl 8:40–57, 1989

Dickson DW, Llena JF, Weidenhein KM, et al: Central nervous system pathology in children with AIDS and facial neurologic signs, stroke and lymphoma, in Brain in Pediatric AIDS. Edited by Kozloski PB. Farmington, CT, Karger, 1990, pp 147–157

Epstein LG, Sharer LR, Joshi VV, et al: Progressive encephalopathy in children with acquired immune deficiency syndrome. Ann Neurol 17:488–496, 1985

Epstein LG, Sharer LR, Oleske JM, et al: Neurologic manifestations of human immunodeficiency virus infection in children. Pediatrics 78:678–687, 1986

Epstein LG, Goudsmit J, Paul DA, et al: Expression of human immunodeficiency virus in cerebrospinal fluid of children with progressive encephalopathy. Ann Neurol 21:397–401, 1987

Epstein LG, Sharer LR, Goudsmit J: Neurological and neuropathological features of HIV in children. Ann Neurol 23 (suppl):S19–S23, 1988a

Epstein LG, Dicarlo F, Joshi V, et al: Primary lymphoma of the central nervous system in children with acquired immunodeficiency syndrome. Pediatrics 82:355–363, 1988b

European Collaborative Study: Neurologic signs in young children with human immunodeficiency virus infection. Pediatr Infect Dis J 9:402–406, 1990

Falloon J, Eddy J, Weiner L, et al: Immunodeficiency virus infection in children. J Pediatr 114:1–30, 1989

Frank Y, Lim W, Kahn E, et al: Multiple ischemic infarcts in a child with AIDS, varicella zoster infection and cerebral vasculitis. Pediatr Neurol 5:64–67, 1989

Gabuzda DH, Ho DD, dela Monte SM, et al: Immunohistochemical identification of HTLV-III antigen in brains of patients with AIDS. Ann Neurol 20:259–295, 1986

Goudsmit J, de Wolf F, Paul DA, et al: Expression of human immunodeficiency virus antigen (HIV-ag) in serum and cerebrospinal fluid during acute and chronic infection. Lancet 2:177–180, 1986

Hittelman J, Fikrig S, Mendez H, et al: Neurodevelopmental assessment of children with symptomatic HIV infection. T.B.P.180 Abstract from the 5th International Conference on AIDS, Montreal, Quebec, Canada, June 1989

Ho DD, Rota TR, Schooley RT, et al: Isolation of HTLV-III from CSF and neural tissues of patients with AIDS related neurologic syndromes. N Engl J Med 313:1493–1497, 1985

Johnson RT, McCarthur JC, Narayan O: The neurobiology of human immunodeficiency virus infection. FASEB J 2:2970–2981, 1988

Kure K, Park YD, Kim TS, et al: Immunohistochemical localization of an HIV epitope in cerebral aneurysmal arteriopathy in pediatric AIDS. Pediatr Pathol 9:655–662, 1989

Kure K, Weidenhein KM, Lyman W, et al: Morphology and distribution of HIV-1 Gp41 positive microglia in subacute AIDS encephalitis. Acta Neuropathol (Berl) 80:393–400, 1990

Levy JA, Shimabukuro JM, Hollander H, et al: Isolation of AIDS associated retrovirus from cerebrospinal fluid and brain of patients with neurological symptoms. Lancet 2:586–588, 1985

Loveland KA, Stehbens JA: Early neurodevelopmental signs of HIV infection in children and adolescents, in Brain in Pediatric AIDS. Edited by Kozloski PB. Farmington, CT, Karger, 1990, pp 72–79

Navia BA, Jordon BD, Price RW: The AIDS dementia complex, I: clinical features. Ann Neurol 19:517–524, 1986

Nellhaus G: Composite international and interracial graphs. Pediatrics 41:106, 1968

Park YD, Belman AL, Kim T-S, et al: Stroke in pediatric acquired immunodeficiency syndrome. Ann Neurol 28:303–311, 1990

Petito CK, Navia BA, Cho E-S, et al: Vacuolar myelopathy pathologically resembling subacute combined degeneration in patients with the acquired immunodeficiency syndrome. N Engl J Med 312:874–879, 1985

Pumarola-Sune T, Navia BA, Cordon-Cardo D, et al: HIV antigen in the brains of patients with the AIDS dementia complex. Ann Neurol 21:490–496, 1987

Resnick L, DiMarzo-Veronese F, Schjupbach J, et al: Intra-blood-brain barrier synthesis of HTLV-III specific IgG in patients with neurologic symptoms associated with AIDS or AIDS-related complex. N Engl J Med 313:1498–1504, 1985

Rubinstein A: Pediatric AIDS. Curr Probl Pediatr 16:399, 1986

Sharer LR, Epstein LG, Cho ES, et al: Pathologic features of AIDS encephalopathy in children. Hum Pathol 17:271–284, 1986

Shaw GM, Harper ME, Hahn BH, et al: HTLV-III infection in brains of children and adults with AIDS encephalopathy. Science 227:177–181, 1985

Ultmann MH, Belman AL, Ruff HA, et al: Developmental abnormalities in infants and children with acquired immune deficiency syndrome (AIDS) and AIDS-related complex. Dev Med Child Neurol 27:563–571, 1985

Ultmann MH, Diamond G, Ruff HA, et al: Developmental abnormalities in infants and children with acquired immune deficiency syndrome (AIDS): a follow up study. Int J Neurosci 32:661–667, 1987

Wiley CA, Schrier RD, Nelson JA, et al: Cellular localization of human immunodeficiency virus infections within the brains of acquired immune deficiency syndrome patients. Proc Natl Acad Sci USA 83:7089–7093, 1986

Wiley CA, Belman AL, Dickson D, et al: Human immunodeficiency virus within the brains of children with AIDS. Clin Neuropathol 1:1–6, 1990

Chapter 7

# Neuropsychological Assessment

John M. Watkins, Ph.D.
Pim Brouwers, Ph.D.
Rose Huntzinger, Ph.D.

*O*ne of the most debilitating effects of human immunodeficiency virus type 1 (HIV-1) infection in both adults and children is the emergence of neurological and neuropsychological impairment (Belman et al. 1985, 1988; Epstein et al. 1985, 1986; McArthur 1987; Ultmann et al. 1985, 1987). Descriptions of cognitive and behavior changes including memory loss, intellectual impairment, and depressed affect appeared early in reports of adult patients with acquired immunodeficiency syndrome (AIDS). These neurological complications were originally referred to as "subacute encephalitis" (Snider et al. 1983) or "subacute encephalopathy" (Britton and Miller 1984) and were thought to be the result of secondary disorders of the central nervous system (CNS) such as toxoplasmosis, lymphoma, or meningitis. It is now believed that in the majority of symptomatic patients, encephalopathy results from direct infection of the CNS by HIV-1, although CNS lymphoma, cerebrovascular accidents, and CNS opportunistic infections may contribute to neurological deterioration (Epstein et al. 1986). These broad constellations of cognitive, affective, and motor symptoms are referred to as AIDS dementia complex (ADC) in adults (Navia et al. 1986) and AIDS/HIV-1 encephalopathy in children (Brouwers et al. 1990a).

We thank Drs. Howard Moss, Philip Pizzo, Katherine Loveland, James Stehbens, and Pam Wolters for their helpful contributions.

# Neuropsychological Impairment in Adults

## *AIDS Dementia Complex*

The clinical presentation of ADC in adults depends on whether the patient is examined early or late in the course of the infection. However, to date we have no definitive longitudinal data on the natural history of the dementia, and we thus have no sure way of predicting who will progress from forgetfulness to full-blown ADC.

The early features of ADC have been characterized by single or multiple impairments in cognitive, motor, and affective functioning (McArthur 1987; Navia et al. 1986; Price et al. 1988a). Within samples of primarily adult homosexual and bisexual males, forgetfulness and loss of concentration have been the most frequently identified early symptoms. The characteristic complaints of memory and attentional impairment have included difficulties in recalling recent personal, social, or medical information and in maintaining full attention to conversations or written materials. Motor symptoms, particularly unsteady gait and leg weakness, as well as behavior changes such as apathy and social withdrawal also appear early. Apathy and withdrawal have been characterized by decreased verbal output, a decline in emotional responsiveness, a loss of interest in social and professional activities, and subdued affect. For numerous patients, these behavior symptoms have been treated unsuccessfully with antidepressants (Navia et al. 1986). During this early stage of ADC, many patients have demonstrated essentially normal performance on routine bedside mental status examinations and neurological evaluations.

A global progressive dementia, characterized by severe memory deficits and deterioration in intellectual and social functioning, emerges during the late stages of ADC (McArthur 1987; Navia et al. 1986; Price et al. 1988a). Psychomotor retardation is often a striking feature in this later stage. Navia et al. (1986) noted that virtually all of their patients demonstrated slowing of verbal and motor responses, with both mutism and akinesia observed in many patients. The apathy seen in the early stages may progress to a state of extreme indifference. Mental status evaluations at this point are usually abnormal, and ataxia, hypertonia, and tremor are frequent findings of neurological examinations.

The course of progression of ADC has been unpredictable, and no specific factors determining the rate of progression have been identified to this point. In some patients, the onset of symptoms has been insidious, whereas in others onset has been abrupt with a rapid deterioration in functioning. In virtually every case, however, the emergence of the noted "later symptoms" has preceded death (McArthur 1987).

Estimates of the prevalence of ADC vary from as low as 16% in some studies to as high as 80% in others. This considerable variability is related to several factors, including differences in the geographic locations and referral patterns at the study sites, differences in risk behaviors among groups evaluated, and differences in the subject selection and diagnostic procedures (Levy and Bredesen 1988).

**Selective impairments.** Recent investigations have attempted to delineate the extent and specificity of the cognitive and behavioral impairments associated with AIDS. Comprehensive neuropsychological batteries typically have been administered to adult homosexual AIDS patients, and their performance then has been compared with groups of matched control subjects (e.g., in Grant et al. 1987; Joffe et al. 1986; Rubinow et al. 1988; Tross et al. 1988; Van Gorp et al. 1989a). Specific neuropsychological deficits have been found within a number of functional systems including language (Joffe et al. 1986; Rubinow et al. 1988), memory (Van Gorp et al. 1989a), and visuospatial and visuoconstructional abilities (Tross et al. 1988; Van Gorp et al. 1989a).

AIDS patients also have demonstrated significant impairment on tests that measure performance under time constraints (Van Gorp et al. 1989a). Motor slowing has been observed on neuropsychological assessment tasks such as finger tapping and the grooved pegboard, and further decrements in performance have been reported when a cognitive component is added to a motor task (Van Gorp et al. 1989b). However, there have been few consistent findings across the various neuropsychological investigations.

Results have been influenced by factors such as the extent and stage of chronic systemic illness in the patients studied, the presence of periph eral disturbances, the introduction of potentially toxic forms of treatment, and the type of tests included in the neuropsychological batteries. Depression may also influence neuropsychological test performance. It is also important to note that the samples used in these studies of adults primarily involved men of above-average intelligence and education and included few minority patients. The generalizability of previous findings to two of the fastest-growing groups of individuals infected with HIV—

minority women and children—is therefore limited until further research specifically involving these groups is conducted.

**Neuroanatomical correlates.** Attempts to correlate ADC with other dementing processes have been ongoing since the initial descriptions of the disorder and suggest that ADC resembles a subcortical dementia (Price et al. 1988b). Autopsies completed on individuals who have died with AIDS have revealed several histopathological abnormalities, including diffuse pallor of the white matter, multinucleated-cell encephalitis, and vacuolar myelopathy. Notably, these abnormalities have been most prominent in subcortical structures such as the central white matter, deep gray structures including the basal ganglia and thalamus, and the brain stem, with relative sparing of the cortex (McArthur 1987; Navia et al. 1986).

Magnetic resonance imaging (MRI) has identified ventricular and sulcal enlargements suggestive of brain atrophy and multiple small lesions in subcortical white matter in patients with AIDS (Grant et al. 1987; Jarvik et al. 1988). In addition, examination of HIV-1–infected adults using positron-emission tomography (PET) has revealed abnormalities in glucose metabolism in the basal ganglia and thalamus (Rottenberg et al. 1987).

**Effects of AZT.** In addition to its importance in defining the parameters of the ADC in AIDS, neuropsychological data have proved useful in monitoring the effects of experimental treatments on AIDS patients, particularly with drugs such as zidovudine (AZT) that are known to cross the blood-brain barrier. Orally administered AZT has been found in several studies to result in improved cognitive performance and neurological function for adult patients with AIDS or advanced AIDS-related complex (ARC) (Schmitt et al. 1988; Yarchoan et al. 1987).

An extensive neuropsychological battery was administered to over 200 AIDS and ARC patients as part of the AZT Collaborative Working Group's large, double-blind, placebo-controlled trial of the efficacy and safety of AZT. Compared with patients taking the placebo, individuals taking AZT demonstrated significant improvements on measures of attention, memory, and visuomotor skills after 8 and 16 weeks of treatment (Schmitt et al. 1988).

## Impairment in Asymptomatic Patients

Although it is generally accepted that HIV-1 is present in the CNS early in the course of the infection (Price et al. 1988b), there is controversy concerning whether neuropsychological impairment occurs in early asymptomatic HIV-1 infection or is associated only with severe immunosuppression. Grant et al. (1987) reported that 44% (7 of 16) of their sample of asymptomatic seropositive subjects demonstrated clinically abnormal performance on neuropsychological measures. In contrast, findings from the Multicenter AIDS Cohort Study (MACS; Selnes et al. 1988) and Air Force (Goethe et al. 1989) and Australian (Gibbs et al. 1990) studies, in which much larger samples of subjects were used, revealed no significant group differences in neuropsychological test performance between asymptomatic seropositive individuals and seronegative controls. However, selective neuropsychological impairment has been found in infected patients before the onset of AIDS, but after marked immunosuppression (Gibbs et al. 1990; Van Gorp et al. 1989a).

At this time, the controversy regarding when HIV-1 has a neuropathological effect on cognitive performance has not been resolved. Therefore, in clinical application, it may not be valid to generalize findings of impairment known to occur in symptomatic patients to asymptomatic seropositive individuals (Van Gorp et al. 1989b). For future research, it is important to note that the group mean comparisons completed in the MACS investigation may have obscured the presence of significant individual cognitive impairment for at least some asymptomatic seropositive persons. Indeed, the contrasting clinical presentations of early versus late ADC that have been described in patients diagnosed with AIDS allude to the possibility that subtypes of neuropathology for HIV-1 infection might exist. Multivariate statistical procedures such as discriminant analysis or cluster analysis allow for the evaluation of individual patients within the context of larger groups or subgroups and thus might prove useful in clarifying this issue. Resolution of this controversy will be important, particularly because of the implications it has in determining when treatment for infected persons should begin. Antiretroviral therapy could be indicated for patients who present with cognitive symptomatology, and treatment early in the course of HIV-1 infection might prevent the development of severe cognitive deficits. Moreover, cognitive impairment and early behavior changes may signal the need for psychotropic medication (Ostrow et al.

1988). Behavioral symptoms in HIV-seropositive adults, including attention deficits and depression, have been successfully treated with psy-
chostimulants, especially methylphenidate, in a limited series of patients
(Holmes et al. 1989; Ostrow et al. 1988).

## Neurodevelopmental Abnormalities in Children

In children, the primary clinical manifestation of HIV-1 infection is often
an encephalopathy characterized by microcephaly, extrapyramidal and
cerebellar signs, developmental delays, and deterioration in cognitive
and motor abilities (Falloon et al. 1989). Indeed, some degree of encephalopathy is found in most symptomatic children infected with HIV-1
(Belman et al. 1985, 1988; Epstein et al. 1985, 1986; Ultmann et al. 1985,
1987). However, the degree of neurological impairment varies widely,
and the course may be static, slowly or rapidly progressive, or intermit-
tently progressive (Belman et al. 1985, 1988; Epstein et al. 1985, 1986).

Abnormalities in development, including delays or regression in
motor and language milestones, have been identified in symptomatic
HIV-infected children younger than age 5 years (Belman et al. 1985,
1988; Epstein et al. 1985, 1986; Ultmann et al. 1985, 1987). Developmental patterns in these children are notable for their heterogeneity, and
current efforts at classification have focused on differences in development within broadly defined subtypes of encephalopathy (Belman et al.
1988; Epstein et al. 1986) or within the broadly defined categories of
AIDS and ARC (Epstein et al. 1986; Ultmann et al. 1985, 1987).

### Progressive Encephalopathy

Children with progressive encephalopathy have impaired brain growth,
loss of developmental milestones, and progressive motor dysfunction
with pyramidal tract signs (Belman and Dickson, Chapter 6, this volume;
Epstein et al. 1988). In children younger than age 5 years, the most
prominent feature reported has been a loss of motor milestones (Epstein
et al. 1986; Ultmann et al. 1985), whereas in older children, impairments
in perceptual-motor function have been reported (Epstein et al. 1986).
Subacute progressive and plateau phases in the course of progressive
encephalopathy have been described (Belman et al. 1988), sometimes
alternating in a stepwise fashion (Epstein et al. 1986). Motor and language skills may diverge during the plateau phase, with motor skills

being relatively more impaired (Belman et al. 1985; Pizzo et al. 1988). Impairment in progressive encephalopathy is increasingly pervasive across developmental domains, gradually leading to deterioration in fine and gross motor coordination, language expression, affective expression, and play. Increased apathy (Belman et al. 1988) or hyperactivity may accompany progression of neurological symptoms. Two studies have reported selective preservation of function in receptive language (Epstein et al. 1986) and socially adaptive skills (Belman et al. 1988) in HIV-infected children with otherwise severe motor and expressive language impairment.

Neurological and developmental deterioration are closely linked to severity of immune deficiency. Although definitions of AIDS and ARC in children have varied, comparisons of children with AIDS and ARC have shown that progressive loss of motor milestones has been found only in patients with AIDS (Epstein et al. 1986; Ultmann et al. 1987). However, delayed acquisition of developmental milestones appears to be present frequently in younger children with both ARC and AIDS (Ultmann et al. 1987).

## Static Encephalopathy

A pattern of continued, but impaired, development has been reported in children with static encephalopathy (Belman et al. 1985; Epstein et al. 1986). In children younger than age 5 years, developmental and intelligence quotients have ranged from severely retarded to borderline, although the quotients remain relatively stable over time (Belman et al. 1988; Epstein et al. 1986; Ultmann et al. 1985). Thus, children with static encephalopathy acquire skills and abilities at a rate consistent with their initial level of functioning, though slower than children without the disease. Interpretation of studies reporting development in children with both progressive and static encephalopathies has been confounded by risk factors that accompany, but are not directly caused by, HIV infection, including maternal drug use, hypoxia, frequent hospitalizations, variations in environmental conditions, and malnutrition.

## Selective Neuropsychological Impairments

Various neuropsychological abnormalities have been identified in symptomatic children, including impairments in gait and motor coordination, expressive and receptive language, and cognition (Brouwers et al. 1989;

Diamond et al. 1987; Pizzo et al. 1988). As with developmental profiles, heterogeneity of findings and wide inter- and intratest scatter are the rule. Functioning is within the normal range in some subdomains, but nonprogressive weaknesses may be observed in other areas.

Two domains of cognitive function that seem to be the most susceptible to selective impairment are attentional processes and expressive behavior. Attention deficits are frequently recognized in children with symptomatic HIV disease (Brouwers et al. 1989; Cohen et al., in press) and are among the hallmark observations in adults with ADC (Price et al. 1988b). In children, attention deficits appear in both relative weaknesses on the "freedom from distractibility" subscales of IQ tests and on behavioral assessment (Brouwers et al. 1989). It is unclear whether attentional symptoms in children are directly attributable to HIV. A number of alternative explanations related to both the medical and psychosocial histories of these children are plausible. In addition, for this age-group, the base rate of attention disorders is relatively high in the general population.

Expressive behavior is also differentially affected. Relatively greater impairment in expressive than in receptive language has been reported in children with symptomatic HIV infection (Epstein et al. 1986; Wolters et al. 1989). Children with symptomatic HIV infection also have difficulty in expressing their feelings and emotions, both verbally and nonverbally (Moss et al. 1989). In addition, significant motor involvement may be seen that is quite independent from the general level of cognitive functioning. These motor impairments may reduce the reliability with which neuropsychological functioning can be assessed, particularly in the very young. It is unclear at this time whether the apparently greater impairment in expressive behaviors reflects a dissociation in abilities characteristic of the effects of HIV on the developing brain or whether this is simply consistent with the pattern seen generally in brain-injured children.

Little is known about neurodevelopment in asymptomatic seropositive children. In vertically infected children (children who acquired HIV through their mothers), there appears to be a bimodal distribution of age at onset of symptoms, including neurological signs (Auger et al. 1988; Scott et al. 1989). Many centers are now reporting vertically infected children in the 8- to 13-year age range who are virtually asymptomatic and who have no obvious neurological symptoms. However, subtle neuropsychological impairments may begin to appear in relatively asymptomatic children many years after infection. In one of the only studies of neuropsychological development in both asymptomatic and symptomatic seropositive children, Cohen et al. (in press) compared 15 HIV-1–seropositive children infected through neonatal blood transfusion to 33 HIV-1–seronegative children who had also received blood transfusions as neonates. Of the seropositive group, 67% were asymptomatic. Although seropositive and seronegative groups did not differ in overall intelligence test scores, small though statistically significant differences were found on measures of school achievement, motor speed, visual scanning, and cognitive flexibility. These children were infected 4–8 years before these assessments, indicating that HIV-1 infection may be followed by years of relatively normal cognitive functioning.

## Effects of Antiretroviral Therapy

Several studies now indicate that therapies that are effective against HIV-1 replication, thus removing some of the HIV-1 burden on the CNS, may also improve neuropsychological functioning in children (Brouwers et al. 1990b; Pizzo et al. 1988). Differences in CNS bioavailability of compounds or their active metabolites and specific effects on neurotoxic cytokines of HIV may result in differential CNS effects of antiretroviral agents. Pizzo et al. (1988) and Brouwers et al. (1990b) have reported significant improvements in neurodevelopmental and cognitive function of HIV-infected children after continuous intravenous infusion treatment with the antiretroviral agent AZT. In these initial studies, almost all patients showed improvement in neuropsychological function, with an average increase of 15 IQ points after 6 months of therapy. In further studies of oral intermittent AZT, 2,'3'-dideoxycytidine (ddC) and alternating ddC/AZT, and 2',3'-dideoxyinosine (ddI), such overall highly significant group effects were not observed (Pizzo et al. 1990; Wolters et al. 1990). For example, as seen in Figure 7–1, when the effects of continuous-infusion AZT in 13 children with P2 HIV-1 infection were compared with the effects of intermittent oral AZT in 12 children with P2 HIV-1 infection, significantly less dramatic neuropsychological improvements were found in the group treated with intermittent oral AZT (Brouwers et al. 1990a; Pizzo 1990). The basis for these differences could be related to the steady-state plasma and cerebrospinal fluid concentration of AZT achieved by continuous intravenous administration as compared with oral intermittent schedules. Although striking, these data

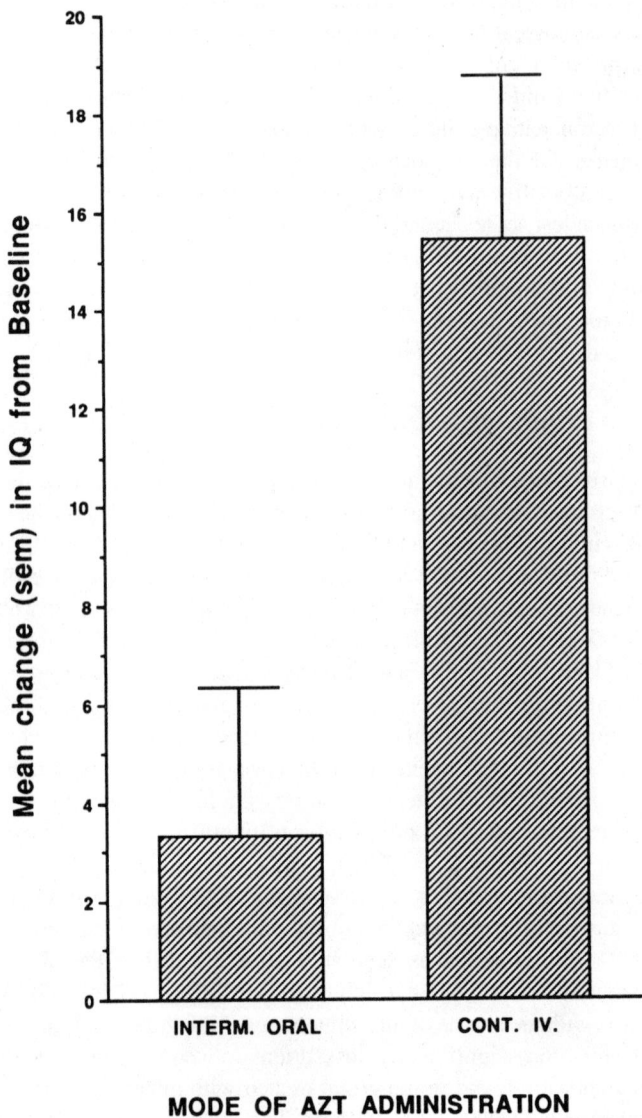

**Figure 7–1.** Change in IQ after 6 months of either intermittent oral administration or continuous intravenous infusion of zidovudine (AZT).

were obtained in two nonblind, nonrandomized Phase I–II studies with no control group, so they must be considered preliminary pending further clinical trials.

On an individual basis, with each of the above-mentioned treatment modalities, some patients have shown remarkable improvements in neuropsychological functioning, well beyond possible practice effects. Other patients have shown no change in functioning or have some documented decline. Because no control groups were available, it is difficult to evaluate these data. Data on the natural history of cognitive impairments in pediatric AIDS, however, indicate either a progressive decline or plateauing in symptomatic patients (Ultmann et al. 1987), but spontaneous recovery in neurological functioning has not been reported. The significant improvements in some children and the stabilization of level of functioning in most of the other treated patients therefore may represent a benefit of therapy. The large degree of variability in neuropsychological response to antiretroviral agents, on the other hand, indicates the need to search for prognostic factors and possible patient subgroups with differential response to these agents.

**Effects of AZT on selective and subclinical deficits.** One of the more puzzling findings to emerge from studies of neuropsychological outcome after antiretroviral therapy has been that even in patients without clinical evidence of encephalopathy or impairment on pretesting, significant improvement has been observed after therapy. Pizzo et al. (1988) found that in an apparently intact group of children with baseline IQ scores within the normal range (81–105), an average increase of almost 15 points (range 8–20) was found after 6 months of continuous-infusion AZT. Minimal deficits noted in these patients were fatigue, depression, and psychomotor slowing. The magnitude of improvement with AZT therapy did not differ from that observed in children with clinical evidence of encephalopathy. These data, although based on relatively small sample sizes, suggest that cognition may be very sensitive to early CNS involvement in children with HIV-1 infection and that subtle impairment in cognitive functioning without clear signs of encephalopathy may be present. A definitive test of this hypothesis, however, will require prospective longitudinal studies of asymptomatic, HIV-1–infected children.

Data from intelligence tests obtained several years before continuous-infusion therapy with AZT have been examined in a few cases of pediatric AIDS acquired through transfusion (Figure 7–2; Brouwers et al. 1990b). In these patients, IQ scores were obtained an average of 4.3 years before therapy, at baseline immediately before therapy, and 3–9 months after therapy. Examination of Figure 7–2 reveals posttest scores that approach the scores obtained years earlier. These cases, together with other data from the Pizzo et al. (1988) and Brouwers et al. (1990b) studies, illustrate one of the more surprising aspects of neuropsychological response to AZT therapy—children on AZT therapy show rapid improvements in functioning that exceed the magnitude and rate of interval change that would normally be expected during recovery from

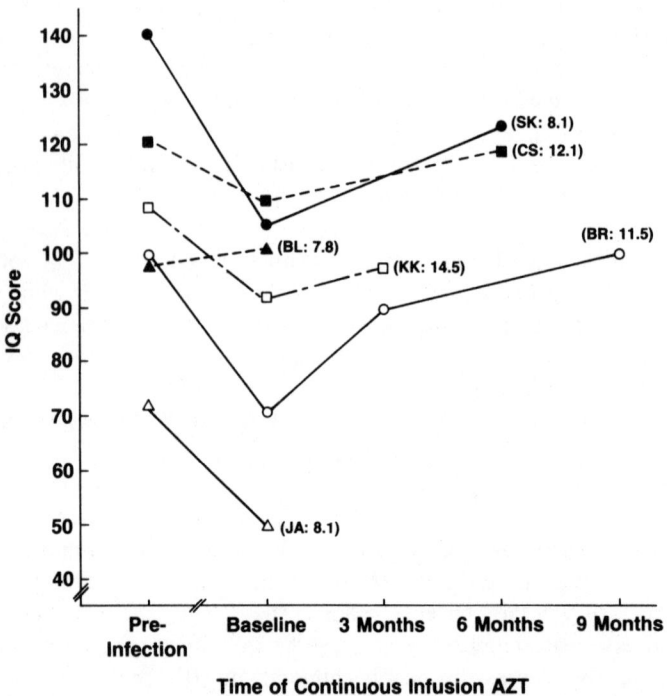

**Figure 7–2.**   Changes in IQ from before HIV infection, to development of symptoms at baseline, to after continuous-infusion zidovudine (AZT) therapy. Letters in parentheses are initials of children. Numbers in parentheses indicate chronological age in years of child at baseline.

serious brain disease. Indeed, interval change after other known brain insults such as head injury or encephalitis follows a slower course that reflects underlying gradual relearning and physiological stabilization and recovery.

This contrast between patterns of recovery from HIV-1–related CNS impairment and other CNS insults suggests that children infected with HIV-1 continued to acquire new skills and abilities at an appropriate rate after infection, but that HIV infection interfered specifically with retrieval and expression of knowledge at baseline testing, at least in children with HIV-1 acquired through transfusion. In combination, these observations support the hypothesis of a specific vulnerability of the expressive components of neuropsychological functioning to HIV-1–associated CNS disease.

In addition to the global effects of AZT on performance on intelligence tests, preliminary studies of therapy with AZT have revealed selective effects on cognitive and behavioral functioning. Moss et al. (1989) found that although children with symptomatic HIV infection showed improvements in general adaptive behavior and intellectual functioning, no change was observed in hyperactive, irritable, or attentional behaviors. This may suggest that either the attentional difficulties are not directly associated with the disease process, or that they are a marker for the HIV infection, relatively unaffected by disease stages or progression.

## Neuroanatomical Correlates

Brain imaging and examination at autopsy have revealed cortical atrophy with ventricular enlargement and widening of sulci, attenuation of subcortical white matter, and symmetric bilateral calcification in the basal ganglia and frontal lobes in some children (Belman and Dickson, Chapter 6, this volume; Belman et al. 1985, 1986, 1988; Epstein et al. 1985, 1986).

In children with HIV-1 infection, there has been only one report of the use of PET, in an 11-year-old hemophiliac boy undergoing a trial of AZT (Pizzo et al. 1988). Pretreatment PET scans of this child showed diffuse cortical hypometabolism and focal areas of markedly reduced metabolism in right frontal and temporal cortex, whereas posttreatment scans revealed only mild abnormalities in the left frontal cortex and overall increased cortical metabolic activity.

# Neuropsychological Assessment Methodology

The unique epidemiology of pediatric AIDS makes it unrealistic to adopt a traditional framework for evaluating the child and instead calls for including larger social structures in the child's environment (Kazak 1989). Neuropsychological assessment in pediatric AIDS therefore encompasses evaluating the child and environment, providing collaborative feedback of assessment information to the family, and coordinating a closer identification between the child's and family's needs and available resources.

## Assessment of the Infant and Preschool Child

Neurodevelopmental assessment involves construction of developmental profiles of children's cognitive, social, and emotional functioning, combined with assessment of their environments. Because children invariably are followed medically over a broad span of development, neurodevelopmental assessment is *longitudinal,* emphasizing multiple assessments across time, and *interactional,* focusing on the reciprocal effects of the child and the environment. A number of recent longitudinal studies of high-risk infants indicate that the health of babies at birth greatly influences the role of the environment on their development, and the environment in turn has an impact on the child's subsequent development. Longitudinal studies of high-risk infants emphasize the need to collect data on social factors in order to understand behavioral outcomes that are a function of the continuing interaction of the infants' biological status and the social environment (Cohen et al. 1986). Thus, understanding the course of the child's development and being able to offer appropriate interventions requires detailed assessment of factors within the child, as well as the child's environmental and social context.

**Components of the neurodevelopmental assessment.** This assessment is aimed at measuring the child's functioning in a number of areas, including cognitive development, attention, social competence, memory, and temperament. Of particular importance in assessing younger HIV-infected children is the attention paid to qualitative aspects of behavior during the assessment process, including task orientation, affect, attention, and activity level. Specific measurement of activity level, smiling and laughter, fear, distress, response to limitations, soothability, and duration of orienting may be as important to the evaluation as the measurement of overall developmental level. Assessment of these dimensions of behavior serves to place the results of developmental testing in a broader context as well as to provide a basis for identifying risk and protective factors influencing the child's development (Rutter 1985).

**Assessment of the home environment.** The home environment has a direct impact on the cognitive and socioemotional development of the child. Extending neurodevelopmental assessment directly into the child's home provides access to samples of the child's everyday behavior and relationship with caregivers and an additional basis for identifying important risk and protective factors located in the home environment. In addition, home visits enhance the collaborative relationship between the treatment team and family, increase accessibility of neurodevelopmental assessment to the family, increase continuity of care for the child and mother, and allow the treatment team to better coordinate the continuum of services that are necessary as the child grows and changes and as the family's needs change. Standardized instruments, such as the Home Observation for Measurement of the Environment (HOME) Inventory (Caldwell and Bradley 1984), are available to assess the quality of stimulation and support available to a child in the home environment. Studies using the HOME with different ethnic groups indicate that the scales measuring parental responsivity and the availability of stimulus play materials were stronger predictors of subsequent cognitive development than traditional infant development scales (Bradley et al. 1989).

## Assessment of School-Age Children

As children reach school age, assessment differentiates to a more extensive sampling of cognitive and behavioral functioning and to assessment across a greater diversity of environments. The primary focus of the neuropsychological assessment is on a valid sampling of functional domains, including language, memory, attention, visuospatial perception, problem solving, and psychomotor function, and secondarily on the specific test instruments used to measure the domains. A second level of assessment is used to relate performance within specific functional domains to behavior within the natural environment, including adaptive behavior at home and at school.

When longitudinal assessment is anticipated, the stability of psychological functions over time also has to be considered because there may be qualitative variation with further development. Thus, developmental changes on memory tasks may not simply reflect increased memory capacity, but may also result from the development of new encoding, storage, and retrieval strategies. Neuropsychological domains relevant for assessment of HIV-1–infected children include general intelligence, language, visuospatial skills, memory, attention, motor function, conceptual thinking, and adaptive behavior. An example of a comprehensive test battery similar to that used in some pediatric AIDS clinical trials (Brouwers et al. 1990a) and in the Hemophilia Growth and Development Study (Loveland et al. 1989) is illustrated in Table 7–1. Testing frequency with this test battery should be limited to minimize practice effects. Due to the easy fatigability of symptomatic HIV-1–infected children, multiple short test sessions may be necessary. It is also often useful to evaluate whether a child can complete timed tasks if given longer to complete the task. Thus, the examiner may choose to be more liberal on the administration, scoring, and interpretation of such timed tests. Unstandardized administration is also necessary for severely delayed children, and it may be necessary to use instruments normally used for younger children. Although this practice does not permit computation of standard scores and percentiles, it does allow for a standardized assessment of interval change in raw scores when tests are administered longitudinally.

**Assessment of interval change.**   Change in psychological functioning in young children is multifactorial. What is meant by "improvement" or "deterioration" has to be defined carefully, because interval change in young children is measured against the force of age-related developmental changes. For example, a child with a chronological age of 24 months and a mental age of 18 months has an approximate developmental quotient of 75, thus showing some delay. After 6 months of treatment, this child has gained 3 months and is now functioning at a mental age of 21 months. The approximate developmental quotient for this child is 70, possibly showing some decrease in standardized performance. Thus, this child has gained some developmental skills and abilities but, on the other hand, could be viewed as having fallen behind the relevant normative group. Raw scores or age scores thus provide a better scale for measuring individual change (Francis et al. 1991). However, reliance on raw score data raises a second issue—many psychometric tests used by neuropsychologists do not provide an interval scale of measurement. Thus, units of change vary at different points on the continuum of test scores, making it difficult to assess growth, decline, and change in scores over time.

Short of designing new neuropsychological tests, a useful approach to more valid assessment of interval change may involve rescaling test scores to reflect an interval scale of measurement. For some applications, Rasch logistics analysis will provide ability estimates in logit units that are interval in nature (Carver 1989), although practical application of this method may be limited to large-sample studies. For instruments that represent interval scales of measurement, growth-curve analysis may be useful when at least four repeated measures are available (Francis et al. 1991).

## Maternal Neuropsychological Assessment

Mothers who are infected with HIV-1 face not only the prospect of having an infected child and of developing AIDS, but also the possibility of having significant neuropsychological impairments themselves. Assessment of the neuropsychological status of mothers of HIV-1–infected infants and children therefore is a crucial component in the overall understanding of the neuropsychological sequelae of HIV-1 infection in the child. To support these women in maintaining their maternal role, it is essential to be able to identify HIV-1–related neuropsychological deficits and to assess and monitor these deficits over time. However, interpretation of test results must be made with the knowledge that the pattern of cognitive test performance may represent an acquired-deficit syndrome or may relate to cultural and intellectual factors long present. Assessment of the pattern of cognitive strengths and weaknesses of the mother assists in treatment planning for the mother, as well as in interpreting the child's neuropsychological test performance.

Standardized test instruments should be used to evaluate these patients. The domain of test instruments from which to choose may be constrained, however, by cultural and language differences between the standardizing sample and the vast majority of women infected with HIV-1. Furthermore, social and economic realities often limit the amount of time that is available for testing to brief periods during regular clinic visits. For longitudinal assessments in asymptomatic patients, a *brief*

**Table 7-1.**  Neuropsychological test battery for pediatric AIDS patients

| Function measured | Test | Age range (years)[a] |
|---|---|---|
| Infant/preschool cognitive development | Bayley Scales of Infant Development (Mental Scale; Bayley 1969) | 0–2.5 |
| | McCarthy Scales of Children's Abilities (McCarthy 1972) | 2.5–8 |
| Infant/preschool motor development | Bayley Scales of Infant Development (Psychomotor Scale; Bayley 1969) | 0–2.5 |
| | Peabody Developmental Motor Scales (Folio and Fewell 1983) | 0.5–6 |
| General intelligence | Wechsler Intelligence Scale for Children—Revised (Wechsler 1974) | 6–16 |
| | Stanford-Binet Intelligence Scale IV (Thorndike et al. 1986)[b] | 2–23 |
| Language | Peabody Picture Vocabulary Test—Revised (Dunn and Dunn 1981) | 2.5–40 |
| | Gardener Expressive One-Word Picture Vocabulary Test (Gardener 1979) | 2–16 |
| | Verbal fluency (Spreen and Strauss 1991) | >2.5 |
| | Boston Naming Test (Kaplan et al. 1983) | >6 |
| Visuospatial | Beery Visual Motor Integration Test (Beery and Buktenica 1967) | 4–17 |
| | Rey-Osterrieth Complex Figure (Spreen and Strauss 1991) | >8 |
| Memory and learning (verbal and nonverbal) | Rey Auditory Verbal (Rey 1964) | >6 |
| | McCarthy Memory Scale (McCarthy 1972) | 2.5–8 |
| | Rey-Osterrieth Complex Figure (Spreen and Strauss 1991)[b] | >8 |
| | Wechsler Memory Scale Designs (modified; Spreen and Strauss 1991)[b] | |
| | Stanford-Binet IV (memory items; Thorndike et al. 1986)[b] | 2–23 |
| | Benton Visual Retention Test (Benton 1974; Benton et al. 1983) | >6 |

| | Test[a] | Age range |
|---|---|---|
| Attention | Target Detection (Reitan and Davison 1974)[b] | |
| | Trail Making Test (Reitan and Davison 1974)[b] | |
| | Simple and Choice Reaction Time[b] | |
| | Continuous Performance Test (Neuchterlein et al. 1983) | |
| Motor function | Bruininks-Oseretsky Test of Motor Proficiency (Bruininks 1978) | >5.5 |
| | Grip Strength (Reitan and Davison 1974) | >5 |
| | Grooved Pegboard (Klove 1963) | >5 |
| | Hand Preference Task (Annett 1970) | >5 |
| Concept formation | Raven's Progressive Matrices (Raven et al. 1984) | >5.5 |
| Adaptive behavior | Vineland Adaptive Behavior Scales (Sparrow et al. 1984) | 0–19 |
| | Achenbach Child Behavior Checklist (Achenbach and Edelbrock 1983) | 2–16 |
| | Videotaped behavior samples (Moss et al. 1990)[b] | |

[a] Age range for which each test is standardized.
[b] Optional or alternative tests.

neuropsychological test battery, combined with a structured interview, is therefore necessary. The battery we have employed is designed to be administered in approximately 30 minutes in each of two regularly scheduled clinic visits. The tests are preceded by a detailed structured interview that evaluates the patient's adaptive behavior in a series of specific everyday environments. The tests for a monitoring battery should tap the major areas of function hypothesized to be impaired in HIV-1 encephalopathy, including memory, sequencing and attention, sustaining and shifting attention, and perceptual-motor skills. A test of verbal intelligence such as the English or Spanish Wechsler Adult Intelligence Test—Revised (WAIS-R; Wechsler 1981) vocabulary subtest may also be administered. Symptoms of depression are also assessed. A more extensive neuropsychological evaluation should be given at baseline that includes assessment of intelligence, language, visuospatial skills, memory, motor function, sensory-perceptual function, executive function, behavior, and affect. Comprehensive neuropsychological assessment batteries for adults with HIV-1 infection are described by Butters et al. (1990) and Van Gorp et al. (1989b).

## Reporting Neuropsychological Assessment Results

Results of a neuropsychological assessment will be understood by the patient and family in the context of broader concerns about the child's or parent's medical care and in the context of the societal metaphor for AIDS (Sontag 1989)—the beliefs, prejudices, and expectations that surround a diagnosis of HIV-1 infection. A finding of impairment on neuropsychological tests may generate frightening expectations in patients, families, and caregivers, including the belief that the patient has thereby progressed one more step in the "inevitable" march toward full-blown AIDS. A closely related expectation is that cognitive impairment will necessarily handicap the patient, requiring removal of the patient from stressful environments. For infected mothers, this expectation may take the form of fear that care of her children will be compromised or that her children might be removed from her care. School-age children may fear being removed from school or placed in a special class. At the extreme of cognitive impairment, the notion of AIDS dementia evokes the terror of a dehumanizing regression of mental abilities that further isolates the patient from contact with both loved ones and society. Like the HIV-1 retrovirus, destructive beliefs and expectations about AIDS can undermine the child's and family's ability to defend and adapt effectively to changing circumstances.

A direct and honest approach to these expectations is to appreciate that, first, we know far too little at this point to predict any "inevitable" course for the infection—especially given the recent introduction of antiretroviral treatments. Second, impairment of a particular cognitive function or skill may or may not result in a handicap or restriction of adaptive functioning. The issue of maternal impairment is especially sensitive, and it is important to remember that there is no criterion-related validity that would predict maternal behavior from neuropsychological tests except perhaps in the extreme, where neuropsychological tests are not needed as a guide. Finally, a host of nonspecific influences including the anger, despair, and anxiety engendered by a diagnosis of HIV-1 infection and the intensive evaluations that follow may exaggerate the perceived impact of cognitive impairment.

## Conclusion: Uses of Neuropsychological Assessment

The unique epidemiology of pediatric AIDS presents major challenges to formulating an approach to the assessment and treatment of children and families with HIV-1 infection. Neuropsychological assessment must include evaluation of the child and the environment, including consideration of preexisting and emerging risk and protective factors, differences in ethnic and socioeconomic environments, and the influence of HIV-1 infection on the parent's functioning. Within this approach, neuropsychological assessment has three broad purposes in the care of patients infected with HIV-1.

First, neuropsychological assessment is used to follow development and, in cases of progressive encephalopathy, to track cognitive and neuromotor decline or improvement. Results of longitudinal neuropsychological assessment may signal the need for treatment, including provision of antiretroviral and psychotropic drugs, as well as measuring neuropsychological outcome.

Second, neuropsychological assessment identifies selective impairments and a pattern of strengths and weaknesses in cognitive functioning that provide a link between the child's needs and specific interventions. Placing information about impairments in the context of intervention and services helps the family remain forward looking and action oriented.

Third, by helping the child and family better understand brain-behavior relationships in pediatric AIDS, assessment provides an important tool for coping with destructive attributions and overly pessimistic predictions about the future. Attributions about changes in behavior that often are made in an effort to explain the consequences of encephalopathy, such as labeling the child lazy or oppositional, can be directly challenged by data from an assessment and by careful consideration of the effects of HIV-1 on the brain and behavior. Modifying attributions about HIV-1 and AIDS and including the patient and family in collaborative feedback about assessment results may have the added benefit of increasing compliance with medical treatment, particularly if patients can directly observe an improvement in test scores after drug therapy. If offered in a sensitive and supportive atmosphere, neuropsychological assessment results can help mobilize the patient and family to take action necessary to recruit and actively participate in appropriate medical care and health-promoting behaviors.

## References

Achenbach TM, Edelbrock C: Manual for the Child Behavior Checklist and Revised Child Behavior Profile. Burlington, University of Vermont, 1983

Annett M: A classification of hand preference by association analysis. Br J Psychol 61:303–321, 1970

Auger I, Thomas P, DeGruttola V, et al: Incubation periods of paediatric AIDS patients. Nature 336:575–577, 1988

Bayley N: Bayley Scales of Infant Development. San Antonio, TX, Psychological Corporation, 1969

Beery KE, Buktenica NA: Developmental Test of Visual-Motor Integration. Chicago, IL, Follett, 1967

Belman AL, Ultmann MH, Horoupian D, et al: Neurologic complications in infants and children with acquired immune deficiency syndrome. Ann Neurol 18:560–566, 1985

Belman AL, Lantos G, Haroupian D, et al: AIDS: calcification of the basal ganglia in infants and children. Neurology 36:1192–1199, 1986

Belman AL, Diamond G, Dickson D, et al: Pediatric acquired immunodeficiency syndrome: neurologic syndromes. Am J Dis Child 149:29–35, 1988

Benton AL: The revised Visual Retention Test: clinical and experimental applications. San Antonio, TX, Psychological Corporation, 1974

Benton AL, Hamsher KD, Varney NR, et al: Contributions to Neuropsychological Assessment. New York, Oxford University Press, 1983

Bradley RH, Caldwell BM, Rock SL, et al: Home environment and cognitive development in the first 3 years of life: a collaborative study involving six sites and three ethnic groups in North America. Dev Psychol 25:217–235, 1989

Britton C, Miller J: Neurologic complications in acquired immunodeficiency syndrome (AIDS). Neurol Clin 2:315–339, 1984

Brouwers P, Moss H, Wolters P, et al: Neuropsychological profile of children with symptomatic HIV infection prior to anti-viral treatment. Paper presented at the 5th International Conference on AIDS, Montreal, Quebec, Canada, June 1989

Brouwers P, Belman A, Epstein L: Central nervous system involvement: manifestations and evaluation, in Pediatric AIDS: The Challenge of HIV Infection in Infants, Children, and Adolescents. Edited by Pizzo PA, Wilfert CM. Baltimore, MD, Williams & Wilkins, 1990a, pp 318–335

Brouwers P, Moss H, Wolters P, et al: Effect of continuous-infusion AZT therapy on neuropsychological functioning in children with symptomatic human immunodeficiency virus infection. J Pediatr 117:980–985, 1990b

Bruininks RH: Bruininks-Oseretsky Test of Motor Proficiency. Circle Pines, MN, AGS, 1978

Butters N, Grant I, Haxby J, et al: Assessment of AIDS-related cognitive changes: recommendations of the NIMH Workshop on Neuropsychological Assessment Approaches. J Clin Exp Neuropsychol 12:963–978, 1990

Caldwell B, Bradley R: Home Observation for Measurement of the Environment. Little Rock, University of Arkansas, 1984

Carver RP: Measuring intellectual growth and decline. Psychological Assessment 1:175–180, 1989

Cohen SE, Parmelee AH, Beckwith L, et al: Cognitive development in preterm infants: birth to 8 years. J Dev Behav Pediatr 7:102–110, 1986

Cohen SE, Mundy T, Karassik B, et al: Neuropsychological functioning in children HIV-1 infected through neonatal blood transfusion. Pediatrics (in press)

Diamond GW, Kaufman J, Belman AL, et al: Characterization of cognitive functioning in a subgroup of children with congenital HIV infection. Archives of Clinical Neuropsychology 3:1–16, 1987

Dunn LM, Dunn LM: Peabody Picture Vocabulary Test—Revised. Circle Pines, MN, AGS, 1981

Epstein LG, Sharer LR, Joshi VV, et al: Progressive encephalopathy in children with acquired immune deficiency syndrome. Ann Neurol 17:488–496, 1985

Epstein LG, Sharer LR, Oleske JM, et al: Neurologic manifestations of human immunodeficiency virus infection in children. Pediatrics 78:678–687, 1986

Epstein LG, Dicarlo F, Joshi V, et al: Primary lymphoma of the central nervous system in children with acquired immunodeficiency syndrome. Pediatrics 82:355–363, 1988

Falloon J, Eddy J, Wiener L, et al: Human immunodeficiency virus infection in children. J Pediatr 114:1–30, 1989

Folio MR, Fewell R: Peabody Developmental Motor Scales. Austin, TX, DLM, 1983

Francis DJ, Fletcher JM, Stuebing KK, et al: Analysis of change: modeling individual growth. J Consult Clin Psychol 59:27–37, 1991

Gardener MF: Expressive One-Word Picture Vocabulary Test. Austin, TX, Pro-Ed, 1979

Gibbs A, Andrewes DG, Szmukler G, et al: Early HIV-related neuropsychological impairment: relationship to stage of viral infection. J Clin Exp Neuropsychol 12:766–780, 1990

Goethe KE, Mitchell JE, Marshall DW, et al: Neuropsychological and neurological function of human immunodeficiency virus seropositive asymptomatic individuals. Arch Neurol 46:129–133, 1989

Grant I, Atkinson J, Hesseling J, et al: Evidence of early central nervous system involvement in the acquired immunodeficiency syndrome (AIDS) and other human immunodeficiency virus (HIV) infections. Ann Intern Med 107:828–836, 1987

Holmes VF, Fernandez F, Levy JK: Psychostimulant response in AIDS related complex patients. J Clin Psychiatry 50:5–8, 1989

Jarvik JG, Hesseling JR, Kennedy C, et al: Acquired immunodeficiency syndrome: magnetic resonance patterns of brain involvement with pathologic correlation. Arch Neurol 45:731–736, 1988

Joffe R, Rubinow D, Squillace K, et al: Neuropsychiatric manifestations of the acquired immune deficiency syndrome (AIDS). Psychopharmacol Bull 22:684–688, 1986

Kaplan EF, Goodglass H, Weintraub S: The Boston Naming Test, 2nd Edition. Philadelphia, PA, Lea & Febiger, 1983

Kazak AE: Families of chronically ill children: model of adaptation and challenge. J Consult Clin Psychol 57:25–30, 1989

Klove H: Clinical neuropsychology. Med Clin North Am 26:592–600, 1963

Levy RM, Bredesen DE: Controversies in HIV-related central nervous system disease: neuropsychological aspects of HIV-1 infection, in AIDS 1988: Clinical Review. Edited by Volberding P, Jacobsen M. New York, Marcel Dekker, 1988

Loveland K, Stehbens JA, Watkins JM: Neuropsychological approaches to the study of HIV disease in children and adolescents with hemophilia. Paper presented at the 5th National Pediatric AIDS Conference, Los Angeles, CA, September 1989

McArthur JC: Neurologic manifestations of AIDS. Medicine 66:407–437, 1987

McCarthy D: McCarthy Scales of Children's Abilities. San Antonio, TX, Psychological Corporation, 1972

Moss H, Wolters P, Eddy J, et al: The effects of encephalopathy and AZT treatment on the social and emotional behavior of pediatric AIDS patients. Paper presented at the 5th International Conference on AIDS, Montreal, Quebec, Canada, June 1989

Moss H, Wolters P, El-Amin D, et al: The use of videotaped behavior samples of pediatric AIDS patients to evaluate psychosocial changes associated with encephalopathy before and after treatment. Paper presented at the 6th International Conference on AIDS, San Francisco, CA, June 1990

Navia BA, Jordon BD, Price RW: The AIDS dementia complex, I: clinical features. Ann Neurol 19:517–524, 1986

Neuchterlein KH, Parasuraman R, Jiang Q: Visual sustained attention: image degradation produces rapid sensitivity decrement over time. Science 220:327–329, 1983

Ostrow D, Grant I, Atkinson H: Assessment and management of the AIDS patient with neuropsychiatric disturbances. J Clin Psychiatry 49 (suppl 5):14–22, 1988

Pizzo PA: Pediatric AIDS, problems within problems. J Infect Dis 161:316–325, 1990

Pizzo PA, Eddy J, Falloon J, et al: Effect of continuous intravenous infusion of zidovudine (AZT) in children with symptomatic HIV infection. N Engl J Med 319:889–896, 1988

Pizzo P, Butler KM, Balis F, et al: Dideoxycytidine (ddC) alone and in an alternating schedule with zidovudine (AZT) in children with symptomatic HIV infection: a pilot study. J Pediatr 117:799–808, 1990

Price RW, Sidtis J, Rosenblum M: The AIDS dementia complex: some current questions. Ann Neurol 23 (suppl):S27–S33, 1988a

Price RW, Brew B, Sidtis J, et al: The brain in AIDS: central nervous system HIV-1 infection and AIDS dementia complex. Science 239:586–592, 1988b

Raven JC, Court JH, Raven J: Manual for the Raven's Progressive Matrices and Vocabulary Scales. London, HK Lewis, 1984

Reitan RM, Davison LA: Clinical Neuropsychology: Current Status and Applications. New York, Winston/Wiley, 1974

Rey A: L'Examen Clinique nen Psychologie. Paris, Press Universaire de France, 1964

Rottenberg D, Moeller JR, Strother SC, et al: The metabolic pathology of the AIDS dementia complex. Ann Neurol 22:700–706, 1987

Rubinow DR, Berettini C, Brouwers P, et al: Neuropsychiatric consequences of AIDS. Ann Neurol 23 (suppl):S24–S26, 1988

Rutter M: Resilience in the face of adversity: protective factors and resistance to psychiatric disorder. Br J Psychiatry 147:598–611, 1985

Schmitt FA, Bigley JW, McKinnis R, et al: Neuropsychological outcome of zidovudine (AZT) treatment of patients with AIDS and AIDS-related complex. N Engl J Med 319:1573–1578, 1988

Scott GB, Hutto G, Makuch RW, et al: Survival in children with perinatal acquired human immunodeficiency virus type I infection. N Engl J Med 321:1791–1796, 1989

Selnes O, Miller E, Becker J, et al: Normal neuropsychological performance in healthy HIV-1 infected homosexual men: the Multicenter AIDS Cohort Study (MACS). Paper presented at the 4th International Conference on AIDS, Stockholm, Sweden, June 1988

Snider W, Simpson D, Nielsen S, et al: Neurological complications of acquired immune deficiency syndrome: analysis of 50 patients. Ann Neurol 14:403–418, 1983

Sontag S: AIDS and Its Metaphors. New York, Farrar, Straus, and Giroux, 1989

Sparrow SS, Balla DA, Cicchetti DV: Vineland Adaptive Behavior Scales. Circle Pines, MN, AGS, 1984

Spreen O, Strauss E: A Compendium of Neuropsychological Tests: Administration Norms, and Commentary. New York, Oxford University Press, 1991

Thorndike RL, Hagen EP, Sattler JM: Stanford-Binet Intelligence Scale, 4th Edition. Chicago, IL, Riverside Publishing, 1986

Tross S, Price RW, Navia BA, et al: Neuropsychological characterization of the AIDS dementia complex: a preliminary report. AIDS 2:81–88, 1988

Ultmann MH, Belman WL, Ruff HA, et al: Developmental abnormalities in infants and children with acquired immune deficiency syndrome (AIDS) and AIDS-related complex. Dev Med Child Neurol 27:563–571, 1985

Ultmann MH, Diamond G, Ruff HA, et al: Developmental abnormalities in children with acquired immunodeficiency syndrome (AIDS): a follow-up study. Int J Neurosci 32:661–667, 1987

Van Gorp W, Miller EN, Satz P, et al: Neuropsychological performance in HIV-1 immunocompromised patients: a preliminary report. J Clin Exp Neuropsychol 11:763–773, 1989a

Van Gorp W, Satz P, Hinkin CH, et al: The neuropsychological aspects of HIV-1 spectrum disease. Psychol Med 7:59–78, 1989b

Wechsler D: The Wechsler Intelligence Scale for Children—Revised. San Antonio, TX, Psychological Corporation, 1974

Wechsler D: Wechsler Adult Intelligence Scale—Revised. San Antonio, TX, Psychological Corporation, 1981

Wolters P, Moss H, Eddy J, et al: The adaptive behavior of children with symptomatic HIV infection and the effects of AZT therapy. Paper presented at the 5th International Conference on AIDS, Montreal, Quebec, Canada, June 1989

Wolters P, Brouwers P, Moss H, et al: The effect of 2′,3′-dideoxyinosine (ddI) on the cognitive functioning of infants and children with symptomatic HIV infection. Paper presented at the 6th International Conference on AIDS, San Francisco, CA, June 1990

Yarchoan R, Berg G, Brouwers P, et al: Response of human-immunodeficiency-virus-associated neurological disease to 3′-azido-3′-deoxythymidine. Lancet 1:132–135, 1987

*Chapter 8*

# The Right of an HIV-Infected Child to an Education

Harold Ginzburg, M.D., J.D., M.P.H.

*H*istorically, the United States Constitution and Section 504 of the Rehabilitation Act of 1973[1] have been used to protect a child's right not to be excluded from school.[2,3] The application of these federal laws to children infected with the human immunodeficiency virus (HIV) who are excluded or discriminated against, in school, has resulted in the children being admitted to the schools. The presence of these children at school has been associated with concern, frustration, anger, and violence in the local populations.[4–10]

Discrimination, by schools, has most visibly affected those children who have the physical stigmata of acquired immunodeficiency syndrome (AIDS) or AIDS-related complex (ARC). However, education discrimination may affect two other groups of children:

- Those who are identified as infected with HIV, but who are currently asymptomatic
- Those who are identified as not infected with HIV, but who either live with infected family members or are otherwise assumed to be at high risk for exposure to HIV (e.g., individuals with hemophilia)

In this chapter, I explore the legal and psychological principles surrounding AIDS-linked education discrimination by presenting an in-depth analysis of two cases. The first case involves the Ray family: three HIV-infected brothers with hemophilia and their noninfected healthy sister and parents living on the northwest coast of Florida.[6] The second case involves Eliana Martinez, a severely handicapped adopted child, with AIDS, living on the northeast coast of Florida.[7–10] An analysis of the impact of the litigation on their lives demonstrates the issues involved in initiating and maintaining an HIV-related education discrimination suit. Both cases were tried by federal district Judge Elizabeth Kovachevich. A review of her cases, from a legal perspective, provides some insight into the application of a complex and controversial medical literature and testimony to the judicial decision-making process.

## Legal Background

Although a state may not be constitutionally obligated to establish and maintain a public school system, if it does, and if it requires all those between certain ages to attend, then the students have a legitimate entitlement and property interest in being able to attend school.[11] In such circumstances, a student has a constitutionally protected right to a public education.[11] The Supreme Court has stated that "education is perhaps the most important function of state and local governments."[2] Thus, any time that a school attempts to deny a child the right to a public education, the courts will apply the highest level of review they can apply—that of strict scrutiny—to determine if the due process clause of the Fourteenth Amendment to the U.S. Constitution has been violated.

The first clause of the Fourteenth Amendment guarantees that no person shall be denied equal protection under the law. This due process clause forbids arbitrary deprivation of fundamental rights. The strict scrutiny examination applies if an individual's fundamental rights are at issue, or if the individual being discriminated against is a member of a suspect class (a class of people who have traditionally been victimized because of their race, national origin, or alienage).[12] Fundamental rights include, among other things, the right to marry (independent of the race of either partner),[13] the right to privacy (e.g., to use birth control),[14] and the right to medical care (e.g., indigents do not have to be county residents for a period before they are eligible for nonemergency medical care at county expense).[15]

Two major pieces of federal legislation directly address the rights of a handicapped child (including an HIV-infected child, whether additionally handicapped or not) to attend school. The Education of the Handicapped Act[16] (EHA) and its amendment, the Handicapped Children's Protection Act of 1986,[17] require participating states to provide a "free appropriate public education" to handicapped children.[18] Section 504 of the Rehabilitation Act of 1973 provides that no "otherwise qualified handicapped individual" shall solely by reason of his handicap be excluded from participation in any program receiving federal financial assistance (e.g., federally funded public education programs).[1]

When a court considers an education discrimination case involving an HIV-infected child, it may elect to concurrently address the EHA and Section 504 issues. The court must first determine the most appropriate educational placement for the HIV-infected (and therefore handicapped) child under the EHA. Then, the court must determine whether the child is otherwise qualified, under Section 504, to be educated in the school, despite being infected with a communicable disease (HIV). The term "otherwise qualified handicapped individual" means that an individual cannot be excluded from participating in, or cannot be denied benefits of, any program or activity receiving federal financial assistance or any program or activity conducted by any executive agency or by the United States Postal Service solely on the basis of his or her handicap. If the child is not otherwise qualified, the court must determine whether reasonable accommodations could reduce the risk of transmission of HIV so as to permit the child to be otherwise qualified to be educated in the appropriate school setting.

The Supreme Court, in *School Board of Nassau County, Florida v. Arline* (1987),[19] affirmed the court of appeals decision[20] that individuals with contagious diseases are within the coverage of Section 504 of the Rehabilitation Act of 1973.[1] Section 706(7)(B) of the Rehabilitation Act defines a handicapped individual as an individual with a physical impairment that substantially limits one or more major life activities. Arline had a long history of tuberculosis. She had been hospitalized for the disease in 1957, and her medical record at that point established that she had a physical impairment (thereby meeting the inclusion criteria in Section 504). The court noted that the fact that a person with a record of impairment is also contagious (infectious) does not remove that individual from being included in Section 504. The Supreme Court noted that the basic purpose of the Rehabilitation Act was to ensure that handicapped individuals were not denied employment (or an education) because of the prejudice or ignorance of others. The Supreme Court stated that the act "replaces such fearful, reflexive reactions with actions based on reasoned and medically sound judgments as to whether contagious handicapped persons are 'otherwise qualified' to do the job."[19]

Macfarlane[21] noted that the Supreme Court, in *Arline*, traced the legislative history of the Rehabilitation Act of 1973 and determined that

Section 504 was created to protect "the handicapped against discrimination stemming not only from prejudice, but from 'archaic attitudes and laws' and from 'the fact that the American people are simply unfamiliar with and insensitive to the difficulties [that] confront individuals with handicaps.'"[19]

The *Arline* Court was insightful in realizing that if it recognized the school board's arguments concerning the firing of Arline, then it would bolster the myths, fears, and reflexive actions that the act was designed to eliminate. Although people still die from infection with the tubercle bacillus, tuberculosis is readily treatable. An individual receiving adequate treatment, for a reasonable period, is not contagious. Therefore, he or she would not pose a health hazard to others. The Supreme Court chided the district court for failing to make an individualized finding of facts about the impairing effects of the disease in question (tuberculosis) and failing to determine how these impairments (pulmonary involvement) affected the individual's ability to participate in the program or activity from which he or she was being barred.[19] District courts need to evaluate each case on its merits, free from community bias and prejudice.

## The Ray Family

The Rays, Richard (age 10), Robert (age 9), and Randy (age 8), their younger sister Candy (age 6), and their parents, lived in Arcadia, DeSoto County, Florida. Richard, Robert, and Randy all have hemophilia of moderate severity. In August 1986, all three brothers were found to be positive for antibodies to HIV; the other family members were found to be negative for HIV antibodies. The three brothers were essentially asymptomatic (from the HIV infection). On August 27, 1986, the family voluntarily informed the school authorities that their sons were infected with HIV. (At this point, it was estimated that 95% of all patients with severe hemophilia were infected with HIV.) The school authorities removed the four Ray children from the classroom; the children began to receive instruction at home. The daughter returned to the classroom when her negative antibody status became known. In February 1987, the father moved the family to Alabama and enrolled all the children in school. When the school authorities found out the boys were infected with HIV, the boys were removed from the classroom. The family returned to Arcadia, DeSoto County, in April 1987. The boys obtained health department certificates indicating that they were able to attend school. The school refused them admittance. Judge Kovachevich, on June 24, 1987, permitted a "separate but equal full-time, isolated instruction" at home, as an interim measure pending resolution of the Rays' request for a preliminary injunction to force the school to readmit them.[6]

The court reminded itself of quarantine procedures that had been used during the polio epidemics, procedures more concerned with the public good than with individual rights. The court accepted its responsibility to make decisions based on the best available, but limited and conflicting, medical information from the authorities. Judge Kovachevich was keenly aware of the studies on the lack of HIV transmissibility among household members who only had casual contact (nonsexual activities of normal household living) with those infected with HIV. In rendering her opinion, she advocated that schools follow the then-current Centers for Disease Control (CDC) guidelines[22] as well as those in the American Academy of Pediatrics (AAP) Redbook (1986).[23]

Judge Kovachevich noted that the occasional episodes of hemorrhage suffered by the children could be best controlled by their being temporarily removed from the integrated classroom, rather than by their total exclusion. Although medical evidence and medical experts strongly supported the Rays' position, an epidemiologist for the school system advocated quarantining the boys, and a physician for the school system recommended the use of "goggles, gloves, and gowns" whenever anyone had to have direct contact with them. Neither examined the boys.

The court allowed into evidence the findings of evaluations of the three boys by an educational psychologist. Each of the three was found to be suffering significant emotional stress, in part, it was alleged, because of their exclusion from the normal classroom setting. The emotional symptoms included anxiety, feelings of rejection, anger, resentment, and fear of social rejection. Bed wetting (where none had existed in the past), crying episodes, nightmares, sleep disorders, and other physical complaints were also reported by the boys. These emotional signs and symptoms should not be surprising, given the strain they were under. It can be readily understood why they felt that they were pawns in a deadly game. The record is unclear as to whether they or their family had access to any mental health counseling during this period. Objective assurance that their responses were healthy would have been a valuable supportive measure.

Judge Kovachevich recognized that the clinical signs and symptoms of psychopathology were directly attributable to the stress of being excluded from the classroom. Her decision was that the actual ongoing injury to the brothers outweighed the potential harm to others, and that the public interest in the case weighed in favor of returning the children to an integrated classroom setting. The court recognized the concern and fear flowing from the small community of Arcadia. Judge Kovachevich stated that the court may not be guided by such community fear, parental pressure, or the possibility of (additional) lawsuits. The judge placed adult responsibility on the three boys for maintaining an elevated standard of hygiene and avoiding contact sports in the school environment and any incidents that could result in blood spills. The judge also ordered the school board to provide education program(s) regarding the realities of AIDS and HIV-positive individuals, the target audience of this education program being the local parents and their children.

The preliminary injunction was ordered on August 5, 1987.[6] Many of the parents boycotted the school, keeping their children home when the school opened for the fall term. Threats of physical violence against the family were reported to the police. On August 28, 1987, members of the community burned down the Ray home. The Rays left the community and moved to Sarasota County. The children enrolled in that school system (without a court order). After a great deal of unsavory press coverage, the DeSoto county school board hired an AIDS consultant (from Sarasota county) to educate the Arcadia community about AIDS and HIV infection. The community refused to attend the lecture.

## Eliana Martinez

Eliana Martinez was born in Puerto Rico on September 15, 1981. She received 39 blood transfusions during the first 4 months of her life. Eliana was adopted in August 1982 and came to Tampa, Florida, with her adoptive mother in June 1983. In December 1984, she was diagnosed as having ARC. In 1987, she was diagnosed as having AIDS and was evaluated at the National Institutes of Health (NIH) for inclusion in a Phase I study of the toxicity and safety of intravenous zidovudine (AZT). At that time she was found to have a mental age of 1.5 years in expressive language and 3.5 years in perceptual-motor skills. Because of her underlying neurological difficulties, it was difficult to determine what portion of her pathology, if any, could be attributed to HIV encephalopathy. Subsequent to the AZT treatment, Eliana appeared clinically improved, but still severely disabled from her underlying disease. The NIH examiners classified Eliana as a trainable mentally handicapped (TMH) child.

In the summer of 1986, Mrs. Martinez had begun the process of enrolling Eliana in the local public school for admission to the TMH program. She did not want to attempt to mainstream Eliana because of Eliana's severe emotional and neurological impairments. The school board had developed an interdisciplinary team to review the circumstances of all children with problems similar to Eliana's. The team recommended, in September 1986, and the school board accepted, that Eliana should not be permitted in the school, but rather should receive her education through the homebound instruction program. Mrs. Martinez objected to the ruling.

Before Mrs. Martinez could commence an education discrimination lawsuit in federal district court, she had to exhaust her administrative remedies. Mrs. Martinez filed her administrative action in December 1986. The evidentiary hearing occurred in April 1987, and the hearing officer of the Division of Administrative Hearings, state of Florida, upheld the school's decision not to enroll Eliana in an integrated classroom setting in August 1987.[7]

Mrs. Martinez filed her first federal lawsuit on September 3, 1987. The complaints were

- Violation of the plaintiff's right to a free and appropriate education pursuant to the Education of the Handicapped Act
- Deprivation of the plaintiff's right to a free and appropriate education in the least restrictive environment pursuant to Section 504 of the Rehabilitation Act of 1973
- Deprivation of the plaintiff's right to a free and appropriate education in the least restrictive environment pursuant to the equal protection clause of the Fourteenth Amendment to the U.S. Constitution

Judge Elizabeth Kovachevich heard the initial motions and all subsequent district court matters. On September 10 and 21, 1987, she denied the plaintiff's motion and renewed the motion for an expedited trial. A motion for a preliminary injunction permitting Eliana to attend school was filed on October 8, 1987, and a hearing occurred on November 6, 1987. Judge Kovachevich denied the request for a preliminary injunction on December 27, 1987.[7] During this time Eliana was being educated at home and was being treated for her progressive HIV infection.

The contention by the school board and its committee of educational and medical advisers was that if Eliana had physical interactions with her classmates she could place them at risk for contracting HIV. Judge Kovachevich ruled that the medical evidence was not convincing, one way or the other. She recognized she was on the cutting edge of establishing new legal principles. This was the first AIDS-linked discrimination case that dealt with an incontinent child. She also was aware of the traumatic impact that her earlier decision in *Ray* had had on the brothers, the family, and the community.[6]

Judge Kovachevich denied the petition for an injunction, on the grounds that the plaintiffs had not carried their legal burden, at that stage of litigation, of establishing the likelihood that they would prevail on the merits of the case. She acknowledged that the actual trial "may turn into a battle of the experts as to whether or not Eliana Martinez poses a threat to the TMH population or whether, indeed, it is safe for her to attend a classroom with other children."[7]

Judge Kovachevich's personal perspective, and the weight of her decision, are noted in her following comments[7] (which also appeared verbatim in the *Ray* decision[6]).

> While we wait for medical science to save us from what many think may be a raging, indiscriminate inferno, it is the task of this Court to deal with the here and now of this lethal, inevitably fatal disease, for which there is currently no inoculation and no cure. The mystery of the virus and its communicability challenges jurists legally to be assured our decisions do not lead us to allow proliferation of this disease by our ignorance.

Judge Kovachevich recognized that her decisions would become the precedent-making cases for others. If the parties did not accept her decisions, as was the case, her decisions would be reviewed at a higher level. If she was found wanting in the manner in which she either conducted the proceedings or analyzed the data, her decision would either be overruled or remanded (returned to her for further consideration). As noted below, the decision in this case was appealed to the circuit court, and they remanded the case.[9]

Judge Kovachevich recognized that the case before her required her to balance the public interest and the potential harm to others. The concept of a risk-benefit balancing test is not new. In 1915, Terry wrote about such a balancing test in his classic article on negligence.[24] Judge Learned Hand made a most notable application of the balancing test in 1932,[25] when he ruled that all available information had to be considered by the court in its determination of whether a party acted properly. A similar approach was used by the Supreme Court, in 1987, to weigh the facts in *School Board of Nassau County, Florida v. Arline*.[19] The elements identified in that case were 1) the nature of the risk (e.g., how the disease is transmitted), 2) the duration of the risk (e.g., how long is the carrier infected), 3) the severity of the harm (e.g., what is the potential harm to third parties), and 4) the probabilities that the disease will be transmitted and cause various degrees of harm.

The Supreme Court, in *Arline*, added that the courts should normally defer to the reasonable medical judgments of public health officials. The Supreme Court concluded that the lower courts must then determine, in light of the evidence collected and reviewed, whether any "reasonable accommodation" can be made to permit the handicapped person to function in the work (or other) environment.

Pollack,[26] in his risk-benefit equation, adds two additional relevant factors that Judge Kovachevich also had to consider: 1) the present ability to predict such likelihood accurately, and 2) the public policy related to the possible harm and to its elements, that is, what is society's response to a given type of harm.

Judge Kovachevich acknowledged these contextual factors when she wrote:[7]

> The public at large has several interests to be considered here. First, is the concern of the public to provide adequate, non-discriminatory education to all the children of this state. The children of this state include children like Eliana Martinez, who, through no fault of their own have contracted this disease provoking in many, fear and a desperate desire to segregate them. However, there is an equally important public interest in protecting the health and safety of the public at large, and here, specifically, the school population which would be in contact with Eliana, if she is returned to a TMH classroom.

A nonjury trial, on the merits of the case, occurred on July 13 and 14, 1988.[8] Judge Kovachevich noted that the CDC, in their 1988 publication *Guidelines for Effective School Health Education to Prevent the Spread of AIDS*,[27] stated that open-mouth kissing theoretically could transmit

HIV from an infected to an uninfected person through direct exposure of mucous membranes to infected blood or saliva. Although she acknowledged a number of studies that demonstrated casual transmission of HIV does not occur, she was most concerned about the risk of infection from students who lack control of their body secretions and excretions.[8] She paid very close attention to the recommendations contained in the Report of the Committee on Infectious Diseases AAP Redbook (1986).[23]

Judge Kovachevich also recognized the need for a team approach in reaching a decision regarding the care and education of Eliana (or any child with HIV infection). She noted that the team should include the child's physician, public health personnel, the child's parent (or guardian), and other personnel associated with the educational setting.[8] She strongly urged that educational and public health departments play an active role in educating other parents, students, and service providers who might interact with an HIV-infected child. This latter recommendation must have evolved from her experience of the results of her decision in the *Ray* case. That case was truly a Pyrrhic victory for all concerned.

By the time the trial occurred in July 1988, Eliana had been diagnosed as having "full-blown" AIDS. Her life expectancy was then estimated at less than 2 years.[8] She was receiving AZT by a continuous intravenous route. Her mental age had increased 6 months in the preceding year. The treating physician in Florida recommended that Eliana needed to be in a "very strictly supervised, restricted environment" and that because of the theoretical risk, "anything that comes in contact with her secretions, should be treated as potentially infectious."[8]

The medical recommendation was that if she attended class, she should be kept at a distance from the other students. The treating physician indicated that he was aware of anecdotal reports that "suggest the possibility of transmissibility by other that [*sic*] sexual contact or direct blood-to-blood contact."[8]

Mrs. Martinez suggested that a reasonable accommodation, under the circumstances, was possible. Eliana could sit several feet away from the other students. She could wear disposable diapers and have her own potty chair in the classroom. She could have adequate supervision with at least three people. Mrs. Martinez noted that Eliana had no restrictions placed on her when she moved about the community at large.

The court recognized the limitations of the homebound education program. The court also recognized that they would be making a medical judgment based on divergent medical testimony. The judge made an apparently gratuitous reference to the Ray brothers in her discussion of balancing the rights of infected students and the community. The effects of that decision appeared to have a major influence on the proceedings in the *Martinez* case.

On August 8, 1988, Judge Kovachevich reached a decision and ordered the school board of Hillsborough County to construct, within the TMH classroom, a separate room of not less than 48 square feet.[8] The room was to have an exterior locked door to the main corridor, a window into the classroom that was at least 40% of the wall, and an adequate sound system for Eliana to hear what was occurring in the main classroom. A full-time aide was assigned to Eliana, and individual parental consent had to be obtained before any classmates could enter her space.

On December 1, 1988, this decision was vacated by a three-judge tribunal sitting for the United States Court of Appeals for the Eleventh Circuit.[9] They noted that Eliana was protected by the Education of the Handicapped Act (EHA)[16] and its amendment[17] and Section 504 of the Rehabilitation Act of 1973.[1] The judicial tribunal reiterated that the EHA requires participating states to provide a "free appropriate public education" to handicapped children.[18]

The lower court decision was vacated because "[t]he record below contains no findings with respect to the effect on Eliana of isolating her with an aide in a separate room in the TMH classroom."[9]

On remand, Judge Kovachevich was ordered to hear evidence on the effects of the isolation on the psychological and educational development of Eliana. The issue presented to the lower court was whether the need for a least restrictive environment was weighed against "any potential harmful effect on the child or on the quality of the services which he or she needs."[28] The appellate court concluded with the remark that placement decisions must be made on an individual basis. (I am hard-pressed to find a more unique set of circumstances than those of Eliana.) However, the objective of the decision was clear. Judge Kovachevich was ordered to take yet another look at the matter.

Judge Kovachevich reopened the case on January 10, 1989.[10] The court took notice of several new medical developments: the revised AAP Redbook (1988) had eliminated the recommendation that "children who cannot control their bodily functions should be placed in a more restricted environment."[29] The CDC published an update, in June 1988, that stated that "universal precautions do not apply to feces, nasal secretion, sputum, sweat, tears, urine and vomitus unless they contain visible blood. The risk of transmission of HIV and HBV [hepatitis B virus] from these fluids and materials is extremely low or nonexistent."[30]

Judge Kovachevich once again referred to her 1987 *Ray* decision.[6] She emphasized that the basic tenet of that decision was responsibility. She had mandated responsible conduct on the part of the three boys and the parents. The court was not disappointed in the conduct of the Rays. However, the court had not concerned itself with the responsible conduct of the community. In the final analysis, it was the community that was irresponsible, throwing all the hard work of the court to the wind like chaff in a stiff autumn breeze. The request by Mrs. Martinez for the school system to undertake an aggressive and extensive community AIDS education program can only have come from her knowing what had happened to the Ray family and realizing the potential for a community backlash against her daughter and her family. Judge Kovachevich concurred in this request and ordered the school to provide such a training program. She too had first-hand knowledge of what happens when a judicial decision is forced on a nonreceptive community.

Judge Kovachevich found Eliana "otherwise qualified" to attend the TMH classroom and therefore found it unnecessary to consider the effect of any accommodation.[10] The decision was filed on April 26, 1989. On April 27, 1989, Eliana went to school and the $10,000 glass cage built for her remained unoccupied. Eliana died November 27, 1989. She had spent only 3 weeks of her last 3 months in school. The funeral procession passed Eliana's school, the school board offices, and the courthouse.

The family believed it was a battle worth fighting. It is doubtful that Eliana ever understood what she had contributed to judicial precedent or that she had helped to guarantee basic educational opportunities for other HIV-infected children.

## Conclusion

This chapter has illustrated the role that HIV-infected children are playing in removing discrimination in schools. They, and their families, are exercising their protected constitutional and legal rights to ensure that they receive the benefits of an education. The battles are occasionally dramatic, always personal, and long and tedious. Those children who have been the center of lawsuits often do not survive long enough to reap the benefits. However, they are making it easier for the future tens of thousands of HIV-infected children who will also want to be educated.

Adequate screening of blood and blood products will reduce the risk of HIV infection to future generations. However, the increasing numbers of children being diagnosed with vertically transmitted HIV infection due to the behaviors of their parents (e.g., sharing of contaminated drug paraphernalia, multiple sexual partners) will overshadow the numbers of children infected from other sources. These HIV-infected children, often from less than stable or intact families, will need to take advantage of the hard-won battles waged by the Rays, the Martinezs, and many others, if they are to have any chance of being as productive as their disease will permit them to be.

# References

1. 87 Stat 394 (codified as amended at 29 USC section 794) (1987) (The Rehabilitation Act of 1973, as amended)
2. Brown v Board of Education, 347 US 483 (1954)
3. New York State Association for Retarded Children v Carey, 466 F Supp 487 (ED NY. 1978), affirmed, 612 F 2d 644 (2d Cir 1979)
4. District 27 Community School v Board of Education, 130 Misc 2d 398, 502 NYS 2d 325 (1986)
5. Thomas v Atascadero Unified School District, 662 F Supp 376 (CD Cal 1987)
6. Ray v School District DeSoto County, 666 F Supp 1524 (MD Fla 1987)
7. Martinez v School Board of Hillsborough County, 675 F Supp 1574 (MD Fla 1987)
8. Martinez v the School Board of Hillsborough County, 692 F Supp 1293 (MD Fla 1988)
9. Martinez v the School Board of Hillsborough County, 861 F 2d 1502 (11th Cir 1988)
10. Martinez v the School Board of Hillsborough County, 711 F Supp 1066 (MD Fla 1989)
11. Goss v Lopez, 419 US 565 (1975)
12. City of Cleburne v Cleburne Living Center, 473 US 432 (1985)
13. Loving v Virginia, 388 US 1 (1967)
14. Griswold v Connecticut, 381 US 479 (1965)
15. Memorial Hospital v Maricopa County, 415 US 250 (1974)
16. 89 Stat 775 (1975) (codified as amended at 20 USC sections 1401–1461 (1982) (Education of the Handicapped Act as amended by the Education for All Handicapped Children Act)
17. 100 Stat 796 (1986) (codified as amended at 20 USC section 1415(f) (Education of the Handicapped Act and its amendment, the Handicapped Children's Protection Act of 1986)

18. 20 USC section 1412(2)(B) (1982)
19. School Board of Nassau County, Florida v Arline, 480 US 273 (1987)
20. Arline v School Board of Nassau County, Florida, 772 F 2d 759 (11th Cir 1985)
21. Macfarlane MA: Equal opportunities: protecting the rights of AIDS-linked children in the classroom. Am J Law Med 14:377–430, 1989
22. Centers for Disease Control: AIDS: Recommendations and Guidelines: November 1982–November 1986. Washington, DC, Centers for Disease Control, 1987
23. American Academy of Pediatrics: Report of the Committee on Infectious Diseases. Elk Grove Village, IL, American Academy of Pediatrics, 1986
24. Terry HT: Negligence. Harvard Law Review 29:40–52, 1915
25. The T.J. Hooper, 60 F 2d 737 (2nd Cir 1932), cert den Eastern Transp Co v Northern Barge Corp, 287 US 662 (1932)
26. Pollack S: The concept of dangerousness for legal purposes. New Dir Ment Health Serv 16:45–54, 1982
27. Centers for Disease Control: Guidelines for effective school health education to prevent the spread of AIDS. MMWR 37 (suppl 2):1–14, 1988
28. 34 CFR section 300.552 (1987)
29. American Academy of Pediatrics: Report of the Committee on Infectious Diseases. Elk Grove Village, IL, American Academy of Pediatrics, 1988
30. Centers for Disease Control: Update: universal precautions for prevention of transmission of human immunodeficiency virus, hepatitis B virus, and other bloodborne pathogens in health-care settings. MMWR 37:377–382, 387–388, 1988

Chapter 9

# The Perspective of Families

Lynn S. Baker, M.D.

*P*ediatric human immunodeficiency virus (HIV) infection is a devastating disease. It is overwhelming a medical and social service system that was structurally and financially unprepared to cope with it. HIV, being a multisystem disease, does not fit neatly into any single specialty or service. Because of this, health professionals who have historically worked alongside, rather than with, one another are having to learn to cooperate in unprecedented ways. Pediatricians, internists, surgeons, obstetricians, and psychiatrists are struggling to learn to work together as genuine teams. Social workers, nurses, and nurse practitioners are having to learn to collaborate with each other in new ways. Government and private research and service organizations are attempting to modify their own bureaucracies so they can behave both responsibly and compassionately when serving families with HIV-spectrum diseases. Caught inexorably in the middle of all this are thousands of patients and families. Increasingly, patients and families are becoming aware that they are being affected by systemic problems that have nothing to do with them and yet affect them directly and often detrimentally.

Health professionals sometimes give lip service to the idea that it is the people who live with an illness, not those who treat the illness, who are the real experts. However, we have rarely included the patient's experience of illness in either our formal training or our textbooks. Nor have we given more than token recognition to the idea that patients—and parents or guardians, when the patients are minor children—should be fully vested members of their own treatment teams (Wolf 1990). Although patients and family members often know nothing about medicine, they know a great deal about the patient, the home, the financial and other stressors operating in the home, and their communities. We know what they often do not: What is *possible*. They know what we often do not: What is *practical*.

One of the consequences of the acquired immunodeficiency syndrome (AIDS) epidemic is an increasing insistence, by patients, that they be accepted as active and knowledgeable participants in all aspects of their illness, from research to treatment to policy. People with AIDS and parents of children who are HIV positive or who have pediatric AIDS are beginning to turn up as invited or registered participants at medical meetings about AIDS in significant numbers, insisting that they belong and that we listen to them. As, indeed, they do and we must (Marx 1989).

They belong in these pages, too. It is my privilege to be the medium through which they can speak to you. What you will read is the result of either formal interviews conducted with parents and children who are HIV positive or have pediatric AIDS or informal interviews and just being a listener at parent networking meetings sponsored by the Association for the Care of Children's Health (ACCH) in cooperation with the Maternal and Child Health Bureau of the U.S. Department of Health and Human Services from August 1989 through February 1990. Those interviews were conducted and the meetings attended as part of my own research for a book about HIV for these children and their parents or caretakers (Baker 1991). This chapter offers me an unexpected and very welcome opportunity to share with colleagues materials gathered in my research that will not appear in my book.

The families who participated, either formally or informally, were from all over the United States. These families were of every sort imaginable: single parent, dual parent, and grandparent; biological, foster, and adoptive. The children were infected by the three most common routes: perinatally, via blood transfusion, and as a result of the use of blood products. None were infected as a result of being sexually molested by an infected adult (Gellert and Durfee 1989). Some of the parents were infected with HIV themselves, others were not. Although the majority of parents were white, middle-class women, all races and ethnic groups, every socioeconomic class, and all levels of education were represented. They belonged to a variety of religious groups and held various beliefs. Given their incredible diversity, it is remarkable how similar their experiences are and continue to be in confronting and living with this illness and its treatment.

If there is one thing that sets these families apart from others with children with HIV, it is their willingness to come out of hiding at least to the point of being there for each other even if they remain largely closeted in their own communities. Whether a grandmother from Brooklyn, an HIV-positive recovering intravenous-drug abuser from Washington, DC, a middle-class family from the deep South, a dual-mother foster family from the Midwest, or a wealthy family from California, each had decided they could no longer handle this alone and reached out to others through ACCH family networking activities. They are the first ripples in a new wave of patient advocacy and awareness of the importance of their input in pediatric HIV research, treatment, and policy.

Whenever possible, I have quoted directly in presenting the parents' perspectives. In general, however, I was forced to paraphrase from my notes as I was not allowed to tape-record most of these meetings and conversations. In organizing the data, it was necessary to simplify and synthesize much of what was shared by the parents. The resulting structure used to present the data vastly oversimplifies the situations and views of these families, but will make their main concerns more clear to the reader.

In addition to the stress that every family with a child who has a catastrophic illness experiences and in addition to the stress that affects all people with diseases for which medicine has no cure, families with HIV-infected children must also deal with another set of stressors that act with something like a domino effect on these families: 1) stigma, which leads to 2) secrecy, which leads to 3) isolation, which leads to 4) lack of support and services. How these unique stressors are experienced and coped with by families with HIV-infected children will constitute the body of this chapter.

## Stigma

AIDS is currently a disease that primarily afflicts unempowered minorities: women, children, blacks, Hispanics, homosexuals, and/or intravenous-drug abusers. This alone would suffice to cause both social disapproval and general neglect of those with the illness. Add to that the fact that HIV is a transmissible virus that causes incurable disease, and disapproval and neglect metamorphose into rejection, abandonment, scapegoating, and abuse. The stories of the struggles the late Ryan White had just trying to attend school were not unique to his community. (See Chapter 8 for similar accounts of children and schools.)

The passage of time and the educational efforts of, among others, former Surgeon General C. Everett Koop have helped partially alleviate the problem of stigma, but it is far from ended (Blendon and Donelan 1988). To be sure, not all communities have vilified their neighbors with HIV infection (Kirp 1989), and the recent "coming out" of a television star and his HIV-infected wife and child have helped raise public awareness and compassion about pediatric AIDS. Even so, the problem of stigma remains. As one mother put it, "When he [the doctor] told me my son was HIV positive, I didn't think about him dying. I thought about what his life would be like as a social pariah."

There are so many examples of the ways that stigma operated that it was most challenging choosing just one to illustrate the pervasiveness and even the subtlety of the problem. As I listened to parents, however, one experience was shared again and again. By its relative simplicity, it may present the problem most clearly.

It was first shared with me by a father, himself HIV positive, as was his wife. Finding a physician willing to care for their HIV-positive children was no easy matter—it often isn't—but that wasn't the problem. What got to him was that the physician they did find insisted that this man's children be seen either first thing in the morning before other patients arrived, or late in the afternoon after all the other patients had left. The reason given for this arrangement was that his children needed to be protected from communicable diseases that other patients might have.

This man is uneducated, but he is not stupid. His oldest child is not infected with HIV, so he'd had some experience of usual pediatric office routines. He'd noticed that, with his first child, sick kids were either seen at certain times of the day or taken ahead of well children to minimize waiting-room exposure. He'd sat next to the families of kids with leukemia who were, he now knew, immunocompromised. He knew that his children were being singled out for special treatment. He had figured out that it was not being done to protect his kids but to protect the doctor, who feared a potential loss of patients should it become known that he was treating a family with HIV.

Had I heard this story only once, I might have attributed it to paranoia. I heard it repeatedly. As this man said, "If the doctors can't handle it—how is everyone else supposed to? My kids are no threat to anyone and he knows that. But he hides us anyway and it makes us feel like shit."

## Secrecy and Isolation

Secrecy and isolation are so closely related that they will be dealt with as a functional unit even though one clearly leads to the other. As a result of a legitimate fear of being stigmatized, HIV infection is nearly always kept a secret outside the family and often within it, especially from the children, HIV infected or not. The parents or caretakers fear that the children, innocently unaware of the potentially devastating response that might occur if they reveal the secret, are better off not knowing it. Another fear is that the children won't be able to handle knowing, or that if they do know they will ask their parents questions the parents are not ready to handle, such as how they got the illness and if they're going to die from it. Although the former reason for not telling is based in reality, the latter is often a projection of the parents or caretakers' own inability to cope with the diagnosis and its implications.

The result is that to protect their children from stigma, many parents lie. They lie to grandparents, siblings, schools, congregations, neighbors, health professionals, and their own children. The most frequently used lie, told to the child and everyone else once a child has progressed from asymptomatic to symptomatic disease, is that the child has leukemia. Before that, they are told vague things like "You have funny blood, like Mommy's" to explain their need for ongoing medical tests and treatment.

Keeping the secret outside the family makes a lot of sense, given the unpredictability of community responses. One black woman, a foster mother of two children with AIDS, lives in a planned suburban community consisting primarily of white upper-middle-class families but that has a mandatory integration policy. She said, "No one knows. If they did, we'd be thrown out. They moved there, like we did, to get away from big city problems. It's a great, safe place to raise kids. Things like AIDS don't happen there. And I'm not gonna be the one to tell them different."

Families who have shared the secret with close friends have lost some of those friendships or had the relationships severely strained. One mother, to get other kids to be permitted to attend her son's birthday party, had to bake two birthday cakes—one for her child, and one for the guests. Many found that their children were no longer allowed to visit other kid's homes, nor were their children's former playmates permitted to visit theirs.

Children with HIV, and even their noninfected siblings, have been evicted from day care and school settings as well as from Sunday school and other religious settings (Kirp 1989; Kubler-Ross 1987; Oyler 1988). Among parents, the advice is to check out a school or school system in advance of enrolling the child to see if there is a written, specific, and nondiscriminatory HIV and AIDS policy in place. If there is not, the word is either to lie or to move elsewhere. When families have taken on a hostile school or school system, been honest about the child's illness, and insisted that the school accept the child, they have always won the legal battle. The cost to them personally, however, has often been so dear that they eventually left town anyway.

One father, years after just such a struggle, was still hurt by his community's response to his sons' illness: "These were my friends. I grew up there. They weren't strangers. They knew me and my family. But they turned on us, acted like they'd never heard of us." He added that, in a funny way, the very people who were demonstrating outside the school his kids were eventually allowed to attend and who were keeping their own children at home would, when they'd meet him one-on-one, appeal to their old friendship to obtain *his* understanding of *their* plight. In the end, he and his family moved to another town, not caring to raise their children in such a community.

Keeping the secret outside the family results in the family being isolated from the sources of comfort and support that communities usually extend to families that have been struck by devastating illness. One mother said, "My husband and I made an effort to go out once a week, to try to maintain something like a normal life. But it was often even more stressful going out than staying home. I'd meet people like you, and you'd all be talking about your kids and your jobs and then I'd get asked what *I* was doing. And I couldn't tell anyone. I'd have to say something like, 'Oh, I quit my job to spend more time with the kids,' and everyone would lose interest. Or, I'd be quiet and people would think I was a snob. The truth was, my life was hell and my daughter was dying and my husband and I could barely stand being with anyone. I'd want to scream the truth, sometimes. But I didn't know how my so-called friends would respond."

The key line of Jean-Paul Sartre's *No Exit* (*Huis Clos*) (1949) is, "Hell is—other people." This is something families with pediatric AIDS know only too well. "We keep [our son's] illness a secret as much as possible," said one mother. "We are terribly worried that if his taboo illness becomes generally known our other son will be viewed as a pariah. We have 'vanished' from the eyes of many friends and from much of society. Our life is far more solitary that it was before this awful period of time began." The use by families of an "acceptable" alternative diagnosis may be helpful, at least initially, to help families obtain the support of their friends and communities.

The secret often isolates the family from its extended family members as well. This was, among those with whom I spoke, particularly true among African Americans and Hispanics, independent of whether the parents were also HIV infected. However great the stigma against AIDS is in white communities, it is evidently nothing as compared with that in minority communities, at least as perceived by the minority families with whom I was in contact. This perception on their part has to be taken very seriously, as these were the families who *were* willing to talk openly, if not publicly, about their disease. One of their biggest concerns was that they felt that there were many other HIV-infected families in their home communities. They speculated that these families were closeted so deeply that they were afraid even to seek medical care lest they be thrown out of their homes and abandoned by the relatives with whom they lived. Just finding these families was identified by their more empowered neighbors as a vital priority—but they also felt that it would be next to impossible to accomplish.

As is the case outside the family, when secrecy is enforced within the family, isolation operates as well. Similar to families suffering from behavioral diseases such as incest and alcohol and drug abuse, maintaining "the secret" becomes the main goal—if unspoken and unacknowledged—around which family life is organized. Because drug abuse is frequently the source of the family's HIV infection, there are often two secrets operating. Family members become isolated from each other. Communication and trust cease to exist just when they are needed most. Individuals get cut off from their own thoughts, feelings, and needs–all in an effort to maintain the secret.

However, just as is the case in families that have become dysfunctional because of behavioral diseases, everyone is unconsciously aware of the secret even if they are not permitted to bring it into conscious awareness or to discuss it openly. And, as with all secrets, it's always only a matter of time before it becomes known. AIDS information is everywhere, in all our media, and increasingly in even elementary school curricula.

In fortunate families, the secret is revealed by someone within the family, usually a child. This can be inadvertent and quite innocent. If the adults in the family can respond positively, everyone benefits. For example, one young AIDS patient was watching the news with his mother. The main story that night was about the AIDS babies in Rumania. After watching it, the child asked, "Is that what I have? AIDS?" With this question, the secrecy and isolation ended. The child and his parents were at last able to talk about the disease, about death—and even more important, about life, love, and hope. In my last communication with this mother, she was planning to attend a parent networking meeting, something she had not felt she could do before.

In less fortunate families, the secret is revealed by someone outside the family, and the result can be devastating for everyone. In one case, the child first heard about her diagnosis from a nurse who said to another nurse in the child's hearing, "Look's to me like that kid has AIDS." In another, the child and her family were in a shopping mall when someone screamed out "She has AIDS!" whereupon there was pandemonium and the shoppers evacuated the mall (Kaplan and Tasker 1989).

Most of the families with whom I spoke had not shared the diagnosis with their children, and all of those who had were white families. These families strongly urged others to tell their children their diagnosis, in simple terms and with a matter-of-fact tone of voice, because they felt it strengthens each member of the family to be able to talk with one another about their concerns and fears. It also empowers the child. For example, one little girl who knew her diagnosis was unexpectedly accosted by a classmate in the schoolyard. "My mom says you have AIDS," the classmate accused. "So what," came the response, "You can't catch it from me." "Oh," said the other child. That settled, they continued playing. The same accusation, hurled at a child who was uninformed, could have been devastating.

Sharing the secret outside the family is another matter, and most parents felt this should be done with great caution if at all. Most of the children who knew their diagnosis were able to keep the secret outside the family. However, there was one little boy who, on his first day of school, announced to his class that he had AIDS. A general panic did not ensue, however, because the child was well informed about his illness and taught the other kids about it. He simply thought having AIDS was something interesting about himself that he wanted to share (Kaplan and Tasker 1989).

To the extent that secrecy offers genuine protection to the child from possible rejection or abuse from members of the community, it is probably advisable and worth the price paid in terms of the family's isolation. To the extent that secrecy offers protection only to the parents, either in covering up their own past behavior or in allowing them not to have to face their own feelings about the diagnosis, it is inadvisable and harmful to the child. A sick and possibly dying child needs, more than anything else, to be able to be close to those he or she loves and depends on. Secrecy within the immediate family serves mainly to isolate the child and make meeting that need impossible. As Binger and colleagues pointed out in discussing the impact of childhood leukemia on families, "The children who were perhaps the loneliest of all were those who were aware of their diagnosis but at the same time recognized that their parents did not wish them to know. As a result there was little or no meaningful communication. No one was left to whom the child could openly express his feelings of sadness, fear and anxiety" (Binger et al. 1969, p. 416).

## Lack of Support and Services

Just as there were no services and sources of support for victims of rape, incest, and the battered-woman syndrome until these problems were acknowledged and openly discussed, there are few community and personal sources of support and often highly inadequate services for families with children with HIV. The oldest community-based AIDS support and service organizations, such as the Gay Men's Health Crisis in New York City and AIDS Project Los Angeles, were established by and for homosexual men, as it was the gay community that was hit hardest and first by the epidemic. Although some of these organizations are attempting to reach out to women and children, their efforts have sometimes been hampered by ambivalence about helping the heterosexual community that traditionally rejected them (Kramer 1989) and about helping intravenous-drug abusers at all. Likewise, many families reported that some organizations that provide services and support for children and families coping with other devastating illnesses such as cancer have denied assistance to their children and even to uninfected family members.

At this time, the number of families of children with HIV is too small to be an effective political force—although certain individuals, such as Elizabeth Glaser, cofounder of the Pediatric AIDS Foundation, have been very politically effective. In addition, these families remain largely invisible and are generally among the most disenfranchised members of our society. They often have little or no idea how to use what power they have or never even imagine that they have any power. They have not yet allied themselves with adult AIDS activists, mainly because of homophobia. As one father said, "I feel sorry for them [homosexuals] and I guess they have the right to do whatever they want. But I think it's [homosexuality] wrong and I don't want to be associated with them." Nor have many felt comfortable in groups that advocate for children with special needs, mainly because they perceive their children as sick rather than disabled and they do not think that parents of children with "acceptable" conditions such as cerebral palsy can possibly understand what they are going through.

As individuals, however, many parents are slowly becoming both assertive and effective advocates for their children–if not for themselves. Their advocacy is largely a response to their perception that the medical and social service establishments don't really care about their kids and view them as hopeless cases—"throw-away kids," as one foster mother put it. "All we hear about is what they may be able to do in 3 years, 5 years. Well, my kid is sick now—and they need to know that they have to do something now."

There are many "somethings" that can be done now, according to parents. Most often identified was a need for greater responsiveness and flexibility on the part of medical institutions, particularly in the matter of parent participation in treatment planning and delivery. One mother said, "As far as I was concerned, *I* was the head of my daughter's treatment team. This didn't make me popular with some of the [hospital] staff, but I didn't care. If anyone entered my daughter's room and didn't introduce himself, I demanded to know who he was. If anyone came in to do a procedure that would inflict pain, I demanded to be told how this procedure would benefit my child. If I wasn't satisfied with the answer, the procedure wasn't done. If anyone came in to do something not involving bodily fluids, such as taking her blood pressure, and they were gowned and masked and gloved, I threw them out and instructed the nursing supervisor that that person was never to enter my child's room again." This mother admitted that she was more accustomed to taking charge and less intimidated by authority than many other parents. Even so, she insisted, parents have a right to make treatment decisions, to have their questions answered to their satisfaction, and to have their concerns taken seriously.

One adoptive mother had great difficulty getting her child's physician to refer her to an experimental treatment program she had read about. "He tried to tell me that it wouldn't do any good, that it was too far to travel, that they wouldn't take him anyway. Well, it *was* far to travel— but they *did* take him and it *has* done him good. His lymphocyte count is back up and he hasn't been sick in months. The doctor is real pleased about it, as though it was all his idea. I don't remind him that he would rather my son had just died than have to go through all the paperwork to get us in there."

Another mother insisted that her child receive all of his care at home. Once he had a central line put in, she almost never took him to the clinic for routine tests. She drew his blood herself, from his catheter, and took it into the lab early every morning. "I think they thought I worked there," she laughs now, "And I wasn't about to tell them I didn't." She managed to get her child's doctor to cooperate with her wishes, and together they found ways to do just about everything at home. Only when her child's status changed suddenly did she take him in to see his physician, and then only for a visit and a revision in the treatment plan she would administer at home.

Other parents have not been as successful as these mothers in obtaining either the support or cooperation of their treating physicians and their teams, especially with regard to home care. This was a major complaint of many of the parents with whom I spoke, and it will become increasingly important as the many HIV-infected parents experience progression of their own disease. They also felt that the physicians who filled in for their regular doctors on weekends or during vacations were often unhelpful, usually because they wanted the child to be brought to the hospital to be examined rather than being willing to spend time on the telephone discussing the situation with the parents. "I could tell when it was PCP [Pneumocystis carinii pneumonia] again," one mother said. "I didn't need a formal diagnosis. What I needed was Septra."

Many parents also complained about the problems involved in obtaining prescription medications after-hours. One mother finally convinced her physician to give her prescriptions for just about everything she might ever need, and she essentially kept a fully stocked pharmacy at home, including narcotics. Obviously, this approach is not suitable for all families, particularly those with members who are currently abusing drugs or alcohol.

Pain management was another problem cited by many parents. They would become utterly frustrated at the attitude of their doctors about the use of narcotics to manage their children's pain. "Here he was, 5 years old and dying, and they're worried about him becoming a drug addict," one parent said. "He was suffering unimaginably and they made this big deal about Dilaudid. Frankly, I would have been ecstatic if he'd have lived long enough to become addicted. You can recover from that." Her advice was not to wait until the child is in pain before giving the next dose of painkiller.

Respite care was another big problem for all parents. Most did not feel that they could hire a babysitter to take care of their child without telling the babysitter the child's diagnosis—so they never hired one. Families without nearby relatives or the means to hire private-duty nurses saw their social and professional lives go down the drain. One couple had not been out together for over 2 years, which placed intolerable stress on their marriage.

Respite care is one area where the organizations that serve homosexual males with AIDS might be able to offer real help to families with AIDS. Many of them have trained caregivers who are experienced in dealing with the management of AIDS. If these organizations set up babysitting services composed of individuals who were themselves not symptomatic from HIV infection, some parents might get a night's or even a weekend's rest from the relentless responsibility of caring for their sick child.

Transportation to and from clinic visits is also often a major problem for these families. Many appointments are missed for lack of either a ride or bus money. This is another area where existing AIDS organizations for adults could help.

Foster parents also identified some problems unique to them, especially the unresponsiveness of the foster care system to the special and often emergent needs of these families. For example, in some areas, the foster care worker, a judge, or even the biological parent has to be consulted before any medical procedure or test, including HIV testing itself in some states, and has to give consent. Time being of the essence in many of these cases, foster parents felt powerless and helpless standing by holding their child's hand and hoping the consent would be granted before the child died. They all wanted more autonomy in making medical decisions for their children.

Another way in which the system was unresponsive was when foster parents sought to adopt their HIV-infected child. In many cases, adoption is a lengthy procedure that can take years. One family learned they had been given the go-ahead to adopt the day after their child died. "These people have to figure out that when they're dealing with a kid with AIDS, there isn't any time. They have to change the way they do things. I'm all for natural parents having rights—but they don't have the right to let their kid die without a name."

If foster parents have a problem, custodial grandparents have an even greater one. They often have no legal authority over medical decisions involving the child they are raising, at least while the parents of the child are alive, while bearing all the responsibility. Their need for respite care is often greater, too, because they frequently have no one to turn to for assistance, and because of their age their own health status is often not the best.

If there is an overall theme to what parents or caregivers feel their needs to be, it is a wish to be taken seriously for the job they do and a wish for more flexibility and creativity on the part of those providing services to them. There is a great deal of anger toward the medical and social service establishments for their lack of sensitivity and insistence on putting their own routines before the needs of the patients and families. Although some of this is likely displaced anger over their own predicament and their feelings of impotence and frustration about their child's disease, much of it is reality based. They are experiencing, first hand, all the shortcomings of a health care system that was so unprepared for anything like HIV that it is only through these families that these shortcomings are being revealed. The most sophisticated among them are beginning to realize that, in their attempts to save their children, they are bringing about important changes in the way health care is delivered.

## Conclusion

The mental health professional who works with families with children with HIV needs to be familiar with several important bodies of knowledge. The first of these is a thorough understanding of the medical aspects of HIV, its natural progression, and all of its manifestations, as well as its treatments and their complications.

The second is familiarity with the way clinics, hospitals, and social service organizations function, so that families can be assisted in obtaining the services they need. Rules, as the old saying goes, exist to be broken—and breaking the rules is often the only way to get these patients' needs met. Mental health professionals need to know how to manipulate the welfare, legal, housing, educational, treatment center, and clinical trials systems. They also need to know how to work with other specialists in being sure that their patients and clients are getting optimal care, both potentially curative and purely supportive, protecting them from being perceived as "throw away" families.

The third is gaining a working knowledge of two bodies of literature, one medical and one popular. The medical literature is that of the stresses placed on all families with seriously ill children. There is a large body of literature on the effects of diseases such as cancer and juvenile-onset diabetes on families and on children's growth and development. An important part of the development of these children is incorporating these conditions as part of their identities, which will become even more important as early treatment prolongs their lives to adolescence and beyond (Blos 1967). The popular one is the body of literature that has been created as a result of the many 12-step programs, dealing not only with chemical dependency but also with how families become dysfunctional when they are organized around protecting a secret (Black 1981; Wegscheider 1981; Woititz 1983). Familiarity with this literature will also be useful in working with HIV-infected children who survive to adolescence, as they will be at high risk for dangerous acting out if they have not already incorporated their disease into their identities. It will also be helpful in working with families in which chemical or sexual addictions preceded or caused the introduction of HIV into the family and in which these addictions may be ongoing problems.

Finally, we need to spend as much time as we can just listening to the lay experts: to the patients and those who care for them. We must design programs that meet their needs rather than our own and be realistic about how these families can and should be helped. We must carefully explore our attitudes toward who these people are and what they are capable of. We must help them provide the best possible lives for their children—and when that is not possible, the most humane deaths. We have to respect and take them seriously if we want them to respect and take us seriously. In pediatric HIV infection, we are all students and we are all teachers—even, and maybe especially, the children.

# References

Baker LS: You and HIV: A Day at a Time. Philadelphia, PA, WB Saunders, 1991
Binger CM, Albin AR, Feurstein RC, et al: Childhood leukemia: emotional impact on patient and family. N Engl J Med 280:414–418, 1969

Black C: It Will Never Happen to Me. Denver, CO, MAC Printing & Publications Division, 1981

Blendon RJ, Donelan K: Discrimination against people with AIDS. N Engl J Med 319:1022–1026, 1988

Blos P: The second individuation process of adolescence. Psychoanal Study Child 22:162–186, 1967

Gellert GA, Durfee MJ: HIV infection and child abuse (letter). N Engl J Med 321:685, 1989

Kaplan M, Tasker M: The child with AIDS. Paper presented at the 5th National Pediatric AIDS Conference, Los Angeles, CA, September 1989

Kirp D: Learning by Heart. New Brunswick, NJ, Rutgers University Press, 1989

Kramer L: Reports From the Holocaust. New York, St. Martin's Press, 1989

Kubler-Ross E: AIDS, The Ultimate Challenge. New York, Macmillan, 1987

Marx JL: Hecklers and protesters liven up a dull meeting. Science 244:1255, 1989

Oyler C (with Becklund L, Polson B): Go Toward the Light. New York, Harper & Row, 1988

Sartre J-P: No Exit and Three Other Plays. New York, Alfred A Knopf, 1949

Wegscheider S: Another Chance: Hope and Health for the Alcoholic Family. Palo Alto, CA, Science & Behavior Books, 1981

Woititz JG: Adult Children of Alcoholics. Deerfield Beach, FL, Health Communications, 1983

Wolf SM: "Near Death"—in the moment of decision. N Engl J Med 322:208–209, 1990

# Providing Care for HIV-Infected Children

*Chapter 10*

# Coordinated Care for Children With HIV Infection

Mary G. Boland, R.N., M.S.N.
Lynn Czarniecki, R.N., M.S.N.
Heidi J. Haiken, A.C.S.W.

*W*hen human immunodeficiency virus (HIV) infection or acquired immunodeficiency syndrome (AIDS) is diagnosed in a child, life is changed forever for the infected child and family. Concomitant with the struggle to come to terms with the diagnosis is the need to receive ongoing health care for a chronic life-threatening illness. The child and family members must learn—some quickly, others more slowly—to navigate the often overwhelming, usually fragmented, and frequently unsympathetic system on which their survival depends.

This chapter is based on our experience at Children's Hospital in Newark, New Jersey, in working with predominantly poor inner-city black and Hispanic families whose children acquired HIV through perinatal transmission. The mothers acquired the infection through heterosexual transmission (50%) and/or intravenous-drug use (50%).

The families share many beliefs about health and illness, effectiveness of treatment, and distrust of majority institutions. Although having cultural roots in the South, many of the adults were born and raised in Newark. Few parents completed high school, and many are single parents living on welfare. Most had heard of AIDS and had some knowledge of HIV transmission but believed it could never happen to them or their children. Once diagnosed, they displayed a sense of fatalism as they struggled to deal with the illness. Extended family and kinship ties as well as belief in God emerged as supports that enabled families to deal with the ordeal that lay ahead. Yet these disadvantaged and sometimes disorganized families displayed strengths as well as weaknesses as they attempted to cope with the diagnosis and care for the child, themselves, and other family members. Any attempt to provide health care must consider the cultural, social, and economic status of the family as well as the stage of illness in the child and the infected parent.

## Classes of HIV Infection

Perinatally HIV-infected infants and children can be well for varying periods, some for several years before developing clinical symptoms. Children are classified with a scheme developed by the Centers for Disease Control, according to their presentation of symptoms (Centers for Disease Control 1987). This scheme, popular with clinicians, will be used as the basis for describing the health care needs of children and, indirectly, the concerns of parents. We recognize that although there are commonalities in needs, each family is unique and must be approached in a manner that acknowledges their individuality and avoids stereotyping. A great deal of cultural diversity among black and Hispanic families is often overlooked or misunderstood (Boyd-Franklin 1989).

When using a chronic illness/developmental approach to HIV infection, it is important to realize that the majority of children with HIV demonstrate some degree of neurologic involvement (Ultmann et al. 1985). In some it is a subtle learning or perceptual disorder. In others it is more profound, with cognitive, motor, and language delays. These impairments need to be considered when providing psychosocial and educational interventions for children with HIV. Because encephalopathy can occur in the absence of other symptoms, abrupt loss of milestones that had been achieved or changes in behavior must always be reported.

Biological parents who are infected with HIV may also suffer from the neurologic sequelae associated with the disease. This may manifest itself as confusion, short-term memory loss, and other mental disabilities. The parent may suffer from a combination of neurologic symptoms, drug problems, and emotional responses to the illness. Neurological, psychological, and social work services need to be provided because the signs of impairment can be mislabeled or go unnoticed.

### Indeterminate Infection

When infection status for an infant is classified as *indeterminate,* the true infection status is unclear. When known to carry maternally transmitted antibodies to HIV and lacking definitive symptoms of infection, the infant's infection status is classified as *seropositive.* Until a definitive diagnostic tool is available, such infants will require frequent monitoring until they reach the age of 2 years (Table 10–1). Those infants with repeated negative HIV antibody tests, normal immune function, and no symptoms of infection associated with HIV are considered to be uninfected. Those whose HIV antibody tests remain positive beyond age 15 months are considered to be infected. During the first 2 years of life, such infants may receive care from a private pediatrician and/or a subspecialist. These infants are rarely hospitalized and can receive care in their own communities.

During the first 2 years of the infant's life, many families use denial as an adaptive coping mechanism. Such conscious denial allows them to continue with daily activities and maintain a normal life. The uncertain diagnosis and wellness of the child permit the family to delay dealing with the implications of the diagnosis. Patient education and referrals for support and assistance may not be perceived as necessary because the family refuses to "think about the illness at all, except the one day a month I come for clinic." During this time, the infected parent may also deny his or her own illness and refuse referrals for care.

**Table 10–1.** Care of the seropositive infant

- Test for HIV antibodies at regular intervals until age 2 years.
- Assess the need for Pneumocystis carinii pneumonia prophylaxis (per CDC guidelines).
- Monitor growth (height, weight, head circumference) and development at regular intervals using a growth chart and tools such as the Denver Developmental Screening Test (Frankenburg and Dodd 1967) or the Bayley (1969) or McCarthy (1972) scales.
- Administer all regular immunizations, substituting killed (injectable) polio for oral vaccine.
- Provide ongoing information and education to the parent or guardian regarding the significance of HIV testing and signs of HIV-related disease.
- Encourage the HIV-infected parent to obtain regular health care. Assess for signs such as fatigue, weight loss, forgetfulness, and inability to follow through with treatment that may have an impact on care of the child.

At the time of diagnosis, families initially experience a period of crisis, experiencing feelings of denial, anger, guilt, sorrow, and anxiety. It is a time of fear of loss and fear of the unknown. There can be disorganization and confusion. Although this crisis can appear to be resolved, more often crises recur with stressful events such as acute illness and hospitalization.

## Asymptomatic and Symptomatic Infection

When the child is known to be infected but has no symptoms of HIV-related illness, contact between health care providers and the child's family is less frequent. The family may receive support, education, and assistance with services on a limited basis. Because the child is brought for care, providers assume that caretakers understand the meaning of the diagnosis and the complexities of immune system function. Frequently, family members are reluctant to ask questions or request information. Other times, they may be overwhelmed with the amount of information provided and have difficulty remembering what was said. Parents require counseling to understand the meaning of asymptomatic infection, the need for regular medical care and prophylactic treatment, and the implications of the diagnosis for day care and school attendance. Some caretakers will be unable or unwilling to hear information regardless of how often it is presented. Denial continues until the family is faced with concrete signs of HIV infection. The asymptomatic stage can last for various periods, with some children remaining asymptomatic until in their school years.

Although HIV infection can be described as a continuum, usually symptoms do not progress in an orderly manner. Many children are not diagnosed until they develop obvious symptoms. This can occur at anytime during a child's life, from infancy to late childhood.

As the child becomes symptomatic, the frequency of outpatient visits increases and hospitalizations begin. This period may be a time of crisis because the reality of the diagnosis can no longer be avoided. Parents begin to ask for detailed information as they again experience a loss of control. The treatment regimen can become complicated as medication, equipment, and procedures become an ongoing part of life. Services can be provided in the home to allow the child and family to continue with some semblance of a normal life. Intravenous medications and high-tech therapies can be safely administered in the home.

One of the most difficult problems that parents and providers face is what to tell the child about the diagnosis, that is, can the child be told the truth. The literature on both child development and life-threatening chronic illness has shown that fear of the unknown is more threatening than what is known—the truth. Although secrecy isolates the child, parents fear telling for many reasons. In such situations, the parent has not been able to adapt to the diagnosis or the parent fears the child will tell others, resulting in increased social isolation. On occasion, professional care providers are afraid and unable to discuss the diagnosis and indirectly support secrecy around the diagnosis.

## AIDS

The diagnosis of AIDS carries a poor prognosis, with most children dying within 1–2 years (Rogers 1988). AIDS may be diagnosed with an acute life-threatening illness, such as Pneumocystis carinii pneumonia, but more often it develops slowly, with progression of existing symptoms such as failure to thrive, encephalopathy, or untreatable opportunistic infection.

The morbidity and mortality associated with AIDS require high levels of service and intervention. During this period, there is great potential for parent-provider conflict, as everyone grapples with the risks and benefits of aggressive, intrusive, and investigational therapies. The family needs assistance to clarify issues and to obtain support for decision making. Disadvantaged families may assume the doctor is always right, not realizing that they can make decisions related to their child's care. The child and family must be active participants in the decision-making process.

## Terminal Stage

Over time, members of the AIDS health care team also develop strong relationships with the family and come to be viewed as a source of support and even as a surrogate family. Care of the child with AIDS during the terminal stage and at the time of death presents the greatest challenge to health care providers. At Children's Hospital of New Jersey, when the child has reached a point after which there is felt to be no benefit to further aggressive treatment, the multidisciplinary team of the physician, nurse, and social worker meets with the family to develop a revised plan of care. Central components of this approach are open, honest discussion of the child's condition, available treatment options, and medical recommendations. This may include a formal meeting of all involved and/or informal discussion with individual staff. The family is encouraged to discuss feelings about the child's prognosis, including their desire for pain management, use of life-support mechanisms, and confidentiality. In our experience, most parents request that everything be done for the child, including the use of life-support devices. A small number of parents opted for palliative care, choosing to keep the child either hospitalized or at home (Rudolph et al. 1988).

Home care for the terminally ill child is concerned with comfort, care, and optimal quality in each day of the child's life (Martin 1985). Hospice philosophy incorporates a partnership between the child, family, and care providers. If hospice is understood as a philosophy, then care can be provided in the acute hospital setting as well as in the home. It pursues the optimum quality of life for the child and family, before and after the child's death.

Often, the goal is not for the child's death to occur at home. Rehospitalization must always be an option (Dominica 1985). In some inner-city areas, community resources to support the family's wish to care for the terminally ill child at home may be nonexistent. Agencies involved with the family such as community nursing agencies and HIV care programs can provide services without the formal label of hospice. Increasingly, home-care agencies provide care throughout the continuum of illness. Financial constraints and safety issues in high-crime areas are usually a concern of care providers. When hospice services do exist, they are an appropriate referral for families. Providers must be cautious about stereotyping families. The parent who wishes to care for the child may be able to do so within the home setting even in the absence of the usual support systems.

Although this chapter focuses on out-of-hospital care, it has been our experience that parents may provide excellent home care and then may choose to place the child in the hospital when death approaches. Compassionate care can be provided when parents and hospital providers have discussed the child's care and agree on a plan. This approach requires ongoing, if not daily, involvement of the physician, nurse, and social worker to assist the parent in decision making.

Families have identified the help of supportive and available staff members as critical during this period. Some families refuse hospice offered near the end of the illness because they do not want new people introduced into their lives. Other families do not share the hospice philosophy. Respecting the value system and beliefs of the family and supporting the family's need for control are important.

The family will continue to need support after the death of the child. For many, the hospital was a very real part of their life. The staff were part of their experience and served to validate the value of the child's life. Some parents have to return to the health care setting because they have other children and some return out of choice, whereas others never return. Follow-up telephone calls and visits are often welcomed, as well as invitations to hospital events. For some it may be too painful to attend, but others speak of their pleasure at being remembered. The death of the child with AIDS presents special problems because of the stigma that society attaches to the disease and to the survivors. Secrecy and isolation have the potential to deprive family members of many traditional supports before and after the death of the child.

## Grief and Bereavement

Grief is a highly personal yet normal response to loss that manifests itself physically, mentally, spiritually, and behaviorally. What people feel, how deeply and intensely they feel it, how they respond, and which coping mechanisms produce relief vary greatly from person to person, even among members of a single family. All of these factors have implications for the types of bereavement services provided to survivors (Boland et al. 1989).

The loss of a child represents to the parent an alteration of the normal life process. It is an aberration. Parents who grieve also mourn for the loss of that normal life process, the loss of their expected future. The child's death foreshadows the parent's own death, forcing the parents to begin to face their personal mortality. Normally, during the time after the death of their child, parents attempt to resolve their feelings, to adjust to life without the loved one, and to get on with the process of living. For the HIV-infected parent, the process of living can encompass both grief for the lost child and preparation for his or her own death.

Caregiving efforts also must address the needs of the surviving siblings who are grieving. Emotional support for siblings must be conveyed with recognition of the differing concepts of death held by children at various developmental levels. Several kinds of emotional support can be provided to various family members, including counseling, support groups, telephone calls, contact with other bereaved families, home visits, and use of volunteers and/or others who have established a close relationship with the family. The resources available to the family will vary because communities are in various stages of response to the HIV epidemic. No one form of support when used alone can be effective in helping the family cope with this loss. We have found that a combination of efforts works best. Offering the family multiple options allows them to discover what helps the most.

As indicated previously, the stigma surrounding the diagnosis of HIV or AIDS can hamper the family's grieving processes, especially when siblings, extended family members, and friends are unaware of the cause of death or do not have permission to talk about it. Caregivers must respect the family's need to maintain secrecy regarding the diagnosis. However, secrecy may inhibit the normal process of grieving. Families will have few persons with whom they can talk openly about the child's death. This may prevent resolution of the loss, especially when the parent, too, is infected with HIV.

Frequently, families seek emotional support from the primary care providers after the child has died. A postdeath or autopsy conference scheduled with the medical care providers gives an opportunity for answering questions about the events leading to the death. Such a conference helps provide closure for the providers as well as the parent.

## Responding to the Chronicity of HIV Disease

A chronic illness or condition is one "with a protracted course which can be progressive and fatal, or associated with a relatively normal life span despite impaired physical or mental functioning" (Matson 1972, p. 801). Such a disease frequently shows acute exacerbations requiring intensive medical attention. The prolonged course and variation in symptomatology require families to deal for years with the impact of illness on the family system as well as the identified "patient(s)."

Although each illness has unique aspects, all chronic illnesses share common issues. The duration of the illness is indefinite but always long, and the outcome is unknown or fatal. Families face the loss of the chronically ill child throughout his or her life, resulting in feelings of chronic sorrow. Often, family members experience physical fatigue and health problems combined with serious and ongoing financial stressors. Even when there is adequate health insurance, other expenses such as transportation to clinics and time lost from work can stress a family's budget. Financial problems are intensified when there is inadequate or no health insurance.

As HIV-infected parents become ill, their ability to care adequately for their child may decrease. The family requires more support to meet the needs of each member. The sick parent may reject outside help in the desperate need to maintain control and to continue to have a "reason to get up each day."

## Foster and Extended Families

In New Jersey, many HIV-infected infants and families are known to child welfare agencies even before they are diagnosed with HIV infection. Parental drug use leading to suspected child neglect (rather than to physical abuse) frequently leads to reporting of the family by health care and other service agencies. In most states, when the biological parent with AIDS can no longer care for a child, child protection workers will try to place the child in the home of a relative. If the parent dies before the child, the child is most often cared for by another family member—a grandparent or an aunt. Thus, the impact of illness may broaden to include an older generation (e.g., grandparents) who have already reared one family and who may not be fully prepared to cope with the needs of a chronically ill child.

In some families, one noninfected member may become the caretaker of several infected persons, experiencing multiple stresses and losses. These extended family members caring for children with HIV infection must also deal with issues of terminal illness, death, ostracism, and stigmatization. The fatal nature of the illness has the potential to affect attachment to the child. Extended family members may be mourning the loss of the child's mother—to drugs, the streets, or death (or all three)—while dealing with feelings of guilt and parental inadequacy because their child participated in a life-style that led to contracting HIV. Frequently, these caretakers are grandmothers who have already raised one family and now must care for a sick child and his or her siblings.

When no relative is available, the child is placed in a foster family or in a transitional group home. Child protection agencies have found it necessary to provide special training, support, and financial incentives in order to recruit foster families for children with HIV (Gurdin and Anderson 1987).

Foster parents have special needs distinct from both biological parents and close relatives. Foster parents need to fully understand the scope of HIV infection, the physical manifestations, HIV precautions, and the special care requirements of HIV-infected children. Foster parents may need added help in the home (such as home health aides) when their foster child is ill or if the foster parent is caring for more than one HIV-infected child. In New Jersey, parents willing to take in HIV-infected children may care for up to two children at a time.

Foster parents must come to terms with their role and the potential for loss of the child. Individuals and families choose to provide foster care to seropositive and HIV-infected children for many reasons. The family motivated to take in a baby whose HIV status is still indeterminate may hope and believe that the child will not be infected and that love can alter the fatal outcome. Others have a desire to rescue the "innocent victim." If the child is truly infected they must face the possibility of caring for a sick or dying child.

Some foster parents have difficulty dealing with their position as the primary caretaking parent while lacking the legal authority to participate in decision making regarding the child's medical treatment. Although they bear the burden of the child's day-to-day care, major decisions such as enrollment in investigational drug trials or halting aggressive medical treatment are made by the child welfare agency and/or the natural parent. Foster families need a great deal of support to care for HIV-infected children. Experience suggests that families with an ability to respond to the multiple needs of the individual child, strong social supports, and experience in parenting are more likely to deal effectively with the stress inherent in caring for the HIV-infected child (Lieberman et al. 1989).

Thus, HIV-infected children live in environments that are possibly deprived and chaotic, peopled with individuals who are highly stressed and psychologically fragile. Although research related to HIV disease and its treatment is extensive, there is little research-based information on the impact of this chronic fatal disease on inner-city, single-parent, poor, minority families or the needs and concerns of extended family members or foster parents. The existing literature on chronic childhood illness has involved research on middle-class families and may not be generalizable to poor families. Additionally, much of this work focused on families with one ill member. With perinatally transmitted HIV infection, at least two family members are infected. There is no comparable model of a fatal illness affecting both parents and children.

Despite the harshness of life in the inner city, when faced with this illness, families do demonstrate the ability to survive. When working with families affected by HIV, it is essential to help them discover the strengths that have allowed them to survive in their environment. Many families can be helped to discover the locus of control of their lives. Encouraging self-determination, self-direction, and self-dependence is important in providing services to people dealing with a chronic illness. Assisting the parent to identify existing problem-solving skills can build self-esteem and help the parent maintain a sense of control. Yet, the daily struggle to meet basic needs can cause families to view health care as a low priority.

## Implications for Service Delivery

Health care providers, including psychiatrists, have to understand that many of these families are action oriented, moving from one crisis to the next with little interest or energy for dealing with psychologic issues in the traditional, ongoing, scheduled, individual therapy mode. Health care services that are perceived as "doing nothing" (i.e., no prescription, procedure, or treatment) are often viewed as valueless. Denial is the most commonly used defense and breaks down only when faced with dramatic signs of illness (e.g., fever, rashes, diarrhea, pain). Therefore, there is tremendous potential for a clash between the values of middle-class professionals working to provide services and poor families struggling and fighting to survive.

The challenge to providers is to engage the child and family by offering services that are seen as necessary and vital. Multiple models for care are being developed in communities throughout the country. Some, but by no means all, incorporate mental health services. Most often, the psychiatrist is requested for crisis intervention during hospitalization or when the parent or child displays such severe symptoms that psychiatric consultation cannot be avoided. Yet psychiatric intervention can be helpful throughout the course of the illness. Various types of intervention including psychiatric assessment coupled with developmental evaluation, group support, individual and family therapy, and collaboration with medical providers for treatment and pain management are needed.

Ongoing psychosocial assessment is needed throughout the course of infection. Social work assessment for abnormal reactions to circumstances and possible referral for psychiatric or psychological services should also be ongoing.

With HIV infection, not only are children and families dealing with a chronic illness but they are also dealing with the loss of peers. Fear of death may be enhanced when children see their friends from clinic die. At times it is useful for the child and family to have one person to work with on emotional issues related to the illness. Psychiatric evaluations can be requested when a child's behavior is considered inappropriate for the situation, such as physical aggression toward staff. Because it is often difficult to differentiate the etiology of such behavior, assessment is requested to develop a plan of care.

Intervention including medication, behavior therapy, and play therapy may be of benefit. Inpatient mental health care is often easier to maintain than outpatient. For many poor families with a chronically ill child, mental health counseling carries little value. New approaches to treatment such as providing therapy at the medical care site, during hospitalization and ambulatory treatment, or even in the home may need to be considered.

To meet the needs of families with HIV infection, service delivery models must be developed that address the issues associated with chronicity and disadvantaged families. The traditional health care models designed to provide either primary well-child care or episodic acute-illness care cannot adequately meet the needs of children with HIV and their families. Health care services can be organized to meet the following objectives of chronic illness care:

- Treat the illness.
- Prevent the illness and the treatment regimen from disrupting the development of the child.
- Prevent the illness and the treatment regimen from disrupting the family unit.

To meet these objectives, the service delivery system needs to be child focused, family centered, comprehensive, and community based. Disciplines providing health, social, educational, and psychological services must work together both formally and informally. Services need to be provided in the home, in school and day care, and in ambulatory and inpatient settings. This requires a commitment to coordinating care either through a primary provider or through case managers.

## Child-Focused Service Delivery System

Any system providing care to a chronically ill child needs to be child focused. This means understanding the impact of chronic illness on children, having providers educated about and experienced in working with children, and having the special needs of children identified within the system (e.g., the need for children to play during clinic visits or in the hospital necessitates play space and child-life workers).

## Family-Centered Service Delivery System

Children live in families. As already demonstrated, chronic life-threatening illness has the potential to disrupt the family. Although children with HIV may not live in traditional two-parent nuclear families, the people who care for them, whether biological parents, grandparents, other relatives, or foster parents, must be involved in the decisions made about the child's care. Caregivers usually know the most about the child, the child's symptoms, and changes in the child's condition and response to treatment. When parents or caregivers are educated about HIV disease, treatments, and care and when they are respected as partners in the child's care, greater compliance and better family adjustment result.

During the early stage of developing a program to treat HIV-infected children, we surveyed parents or guardians regarding their needs. Most asked for a group for parents and requested information on HIV disease and its effect on their children and themselves. However, most could not attend such sessions unless transportation and day care were made available. Parents expressed a preference for meeting around social events rather than a "support" group setting. When offered group social activities, such as zoo trips, holiday parties, and picnics, we found that the families were more likely to attend. These events served as a focus for development of an informal parent support system. Hospitalization and clinic visits provide shared experiences that also resulted in formation of support networks that are ongoing and parent driven. A similar assessment completed by parents of children receiving investigational therapy at the National Institutes of Health, a research setting where parents are highly motivated, found that parents wanted information related to the disease and its treatment and assistance with disclosure of the diagnosis to family and friends. Parents were also interested in a range of counseling services, including financial counseling (Falloon et al. 1989).

Families in the AIDS program at Boston City Hospital were interviewed to define family stressors and perception of positive and negative nursing interventions. Frequently identified stressors included recurrent illness in the child, coping with anticipatory loss, loneliness, and loss of control and normalcy. Families reported feeling overwhelmed interacting with a large number of health care providers. Parents saw the most positive nursing interventions as those that included attention to normal care needs, comfort measures, response to parental concerns and the child's unique likes and dislikes, facilitation of the parent in the comforting role, and the provision of a consistent health care provider. Negative interventions were identified as providers who reflected a judgmental attitude and imposed parental guilt, lack of response to parental concerns, and discomfort with negative emotion (Schwartz 1989).

## Comprehensive Service Delivery System

Chronic illness affects not only the child's physical condition but also his or her psychosocial and family functioning, requiring a service delivery system able to meet physical needs and psychosocial and family needs. A team consisting of physicians, social workers, and nurses is best able to provide comprehensive care. Nurses play a crucial role in the coordination of health care services, health education of parents, follow-up of medical problems, discharge planning, and communication with other providers. Social workers provide direct emotional support, crisis intervention, and assistance in accessing financial and community services.

Children with HIV require the care of almost every pediatric subspecialist. When possible, these physicians should be available within the same system where HIV care is given. Nutritionists need to be part of both the inpatient and ambulatory team. Routine evaluations of development and neurologic functioning require the services of neurologists and psychologists. Physical, occupational, and speech therapists need to be incorporated into the care system also.

## Community-Based Service Delivery System

Community health nurses can become the consistent link with the family by delivering high-tech care, reinforcing teaching, and providing emotional support. Many community nursing agencies provide other home-based services such as home health aides, therapists, nutritionists, and social workers. With their intimate knowledge of their own communities, these agencies can become a vital part of providing care for individuals infected with HIV.

Children with HIV need to socialize with children their own age and to enjoy educational experiences like healthy children. Admission of children with HIV into day care, early-intervention programs, preschool, and school requires special assistance. Principals, teachers, and school nurses need information about HIV and a full understanding of the needs of infected children (Haiken et al. 1991). After appropriate education, school staff can be extremely helpful and supportive.

The multiple problems facing many families affected by HIV also require good communication with community social agencies such as welfare, social security, housing and shelter organizations, emergency food pantries, comunity mental health services, church groups, and volunteer organizations. Health care providers can work to develop different systems for maintaining close working relationships with community agencies. Liaisons, coalitions, committees, and consultation are all ways to achieve the goal of community-based care.

### Coordinated Service Delivery System

The numerous services needed by these families necessitate a high degree of coordination. Without it, some services can be easily duplicated, whereas other needs go unmet. The family benefits from the assistance of one designated individual working to help them obtain needed services. A case management system can be effective, as can the system of having a primary provider act as coordinator of services. Various models can be used provided that family participation is viewed as vital to the process.

The mental health services available will vary with the setting. Using a case management model, the social worker is often directed toward crisis intervention, ongoing support, concrete services, and bereavement counseling. It is essential that health care professionals understand the limitations of their role within their institution and provide referrals when appropriate.

## Summary

As increasing numbers of children infected with HIV are identified and supportive treatment improves, it is expected that the majority of services provided to HIV-infected children will be both home and hospital based.

Our experience at Children's Hospital of New Jersey has shown that—
with appropriate education and support—compassionate and coordinated
care can be delivered to the child and family with HIV infection. Delivery of such care is most effective when provided by multiple disciplines
working as a team committed to the delivery of comprehensive care.

# References

Bayley N: Bayley Scales of Infant Development. San Antonio, TX, Psychological
    Corporation, 1969
Boland M, Mahan-Rudolph P, Evans P: Special issues in the care of the child with
    HIV infection/AIDS, in Pediatric Hospice Care: What Helps. Edited by
    Martin BB. Los Angeles, CA, Children's Hospital, 1989, pp 116–144
Boyd-Franklin N: Black Families in Therapy: A Multisystems Approach. New
    York, Guilford, 1989, pp 3–24
Centers for Disease Control: Classification system for human immunodeficiency
    virus infection in children under 13 years of age. MMWR 36:225–330, 1987
Dominica Mother Frances: Helen House: a hospice for children, in Hospice
    Approaches to Pediatric Care. Edited by Corr C, Corr D. New York, WB
    Saunders, 1985, pp 107–126
Falloon J, Eddy J, Wiener L, et al: Human immunodeficiency virus infection in
    children. J Pediatr 114:1–30, 1989
Frankenburg WK, Dodds JB: The Denver Developmental Screening Test. J Pediatr
    71:181–191, 1967
Gurdin P, Anderson G: Quality care for ill children: AIDS specialized foster family
    homes. Child Welfare 66:291–302, 1987
Haiken H, Hernandez M, Mintz M, et al: School-aged HIV-infected children and
    access to education. Pediatric AIDS and HIV Infection: Fetus to Adolescent
    2:74–79, 1991
Lieberman A, Grosz J, Hopkins K, et al: Paper presented at the 5th National
    Pediatric AIDS Conference, Los Angeles, CA, September 1989
Martin B: Home care for terminally ill children and their families, in Hospice
    Approaches to Pediatric Care. Edited by Corr C, Corr D. New York, WB
    Saunders, 1985, pp 65–86
Matson A: Long-term physical illness in childhood: a challenge to psychosocial
    adaptation. Pediatrics 50:801–811, 1972
McCarthy D: McCarthy Scales of Children's Abilities. San Antonio, TX, Psycho-
    logical Corporation, 1972
Rogers M: Pediatric HIV infection: epidemiology, etiopathogenesis, and trans-
    mission. Pediatr Ann 17:324–330, 1988

Rudolph P, Boland M, Connor E, et al: Paper presented at the 4th International Conference on AIDS, Stockholm, Sweden, June 1988

Schwartz T: Caring for the HIV positive child, the identification of family stressors to target and improve nursing interventions. Presented at the 5th National Pediatric AIDS Conference, Los Angeles, CA, September 1989

Ultmann M, Belman A, Ruff H, et al: Developmental abnormalities in infants and children with acquired immune deficiency syndrome (AIDS) and AIDS related complex. Dev Med Child Neurol 27:563–571, 1985

*Chapter 11*

# Development and Use of Community Resources in Caring for HIV-Positive Mothers and Infants

Toni Cabat, M.S.W.
The Reverend Ross B. Hildebrand, S.T.B.
Lucretia Robertson

*M*others and infants infected with the human immunodeficiency virus (HIV) represent a population, with special needs requiring comprehensive psychosocial interventions and community resources to promote engagement in and compliance with the health care system. These interventions and resources must serve to assist in promoting family stability in the community, as well. HIV infection accentuates isolation, poor self-concept, and social stigmatism for this population of women and children. Diagnosis with HIV adds to their sense of alienation, helplessness, shame, and marginality.

The social configuration of HIV-infected women and infants is partially documented by Centers for Disease Control (CDC) cumulative data and recent literature describing the end stage of HIV illness—acquired immunodeficiency syndrome (AIDS) (Dokecki et al. 1989; Honey 1988; Lewert 1988). On a national level, diagnosed cases of pediatric AIDS show an annual increase of 40%, with 80% of the cases

We acknowledge the support and encouragement of Albert Einstein College of Medicine, Bronx, New York; St. Peter's Episcopal Church, Bronx, New York; St. Luke's Episcopal Church, Montclair, New Jersey; and Memorial Sloan-Kettering Cancer Center, New York, New York. The funding sources that made this work possible are Robert Wood Johnson Foundation Grant 10810 and the Department of Health and Human Services, Public Health Service, Bureau of Maternal and Child Health, Pediatric AIDS Demonstration Project.

resulting from perinatal transmission (Centers for Disease Control 1990). Currently, women (ages 24–35) make up 20% of all AIDS cases in New York City (New York City Department of Health 1989). HIV-infected mothers are passing the virus to their unborn child at a rate of 25–40%. Although data describing the far greater pool of patients—HIV infected but asymptomatic—are not documented, we can extrapolate from cases of AIDS diagnosed in urban cities, like New York, Newark, and Miami, that the population of HIV-infected women of childbearing age and perinatally infected infants is increasing. Infants infected perinatally are born into families where one or more family members are already infected with HIV because the mother has been infected generally through her own drug use (sharing of drug paraphernalia with HIV-infected persons) or through heterosexual contact with an HIV-infected partner.

It is not unusual to have more than one HIV-infected child in a family. Infants who escape infection may indeed be free of this deadly virus but may still be orphaned when one or both parents die with AIDS. The social configuration for this mother-infant dyad thus often includes a family system of drug use or loss of multiple family members, which is compounded by racial and economic barriers.

The CDC reports that 54% of pediatric AIDS patients in the United States are black or Hispanic (Honey 1988). However, in New York City, 90% of the children diagnosed with AIDS are from black or Hispanic families (New York City Department of Health 1989). Poverty is the companion to HIV infection for a preponderance of infected families. In a 1987 paper to the American Public Health Association, Moore et al. reported on one municipal hospital in which 75% of its AIDS patients are eligible for Medicaid (Shernoff 1990).

Denial of diagnosis, depression, rage, and withdrawal from the health care system are common responses. Early medical intervention can now slow the progress of the disease and thus prevent and delay symptomatology and recurrence. Interventions can be prescribed to combat concomitant neurological involvement for developmentally delayed infants (see Chapters 6 and 7, this volume). Early social intervention allows stabilization of the individual and family in the community before the onset of symptoms. The challenge to health care professionals is to overcome the psychosocial barriers so as to enlist and maintain family members in treatment. Traditional interventions from major medical centers, which do not include outreach and practical assistance, have had limited success with this population. Our poor rate of success in enrolling women in prenatal care in New York City demonstrates the difficult challenges presented by poor pregnant women. Therefore, to encourage early identification and treatment of women and infants with HIV infection, the medical center must work creatively and conjointly with a wide range of community resources to develop specialized programs.

The primary focus of this chapter is to demonstrate the range of community support services indicated and the development and use of community resources, principally religious-based organizations, as a means of assisting HIV-infected women and children. The underlying psychosocial issues or recurring themes presented by this population—social and emotional isolation, poor self-concept, and social stigmatization—are addressed through the creative development of a support network, advocacy, and positive reinforcement offered by a wide range of traditional and nontraditional adjunctive services. An interactive model is provided for medical centers and community agencies and institutions. This successful model program reflects the mobilization of community resources responding to the HIV epidemic in a minority population. The medical center is located in Bronx, New York, where some of the highest rates of perinatal transmission of HIV are experienced, but the model is applicable to most centers serving minority women, children, and families.

## Psychosocial Issues—Recurring Themes

### Social and Emotional Isolation

Social and emotional isolation are two of the most poignant features of HIV-infected women and their families. The isolation, whether self-imposed (as a function of fear of rejection, or fear of sharing their "shameful secret" of infection) or imposed by environmental factors and poverty (Garbarino and Sherman 1980), is compounded by the natural isolation experienced by homebound mothers with young children.

The social isolation experienced by mothers of young children in more functional communities is overcome by the development of social networks. Mothers all come out of their homes or apartments with strollers and sit in neighborhood parks. Natural networks develop from their "park friends" in the form of exchange of babysitting services, parenting tips, and much needed social contact with another adult.

Without these natural support networks, and with the added burden of the diagnosis of HIV infection, mothers and their young children remain an unwanted distance from others. Because so many choose not to tell their few friends and family members of the diagnosis, they remain alone in their meager apartments. For example,

> Frances, a young black mother with a history of alcohol and drug use, cried bitterly one day in clinic about her isolation. After a history of repeated abortions and miscarriages, she had given birth prematurely to a son. She learned of her HIV-positive status shortly before delivery. She told no one of her status because she feared rejection by her one minimal support, her alcoholic mother. She also feared the removal of her child by the child welfare authorities. When she came to clinic, she cried out in pain because of the very lonely position her status left her and her son in.

This mother suffered not only social isolation but emotional isolation, expressing "the painful loneliness caused by the loss or absence of a specific attachment to a loved person" (Germain and Gitterman 1980, p. 175). At least when in clinic, she could be comforted by others when she cried. Some women eventually overcome the emotional isolation by taking the risk of sharing their secret of infection with their partner or spouse, mother, or sister. However, before taking the risk of exposing themselves to rejection, they agonize in their loneliness.

## Poor Self-concept

Without the mirror of social and emotional connection, it is difficult for HIV-infected women to maintain any sense of self-concept and dignity. Self-esteem is part of one's self-concept; it allows people some degree of psychic comfort in trusting oneself and others in coping in stressful situations. Germain and Gitterman see individuals as attaining "some minimal control over such threatening affects as grief, rage, shame, guilt and despair" through their self-esteem (Germain and Gitterman 1980, p. 100). Bloom (1980, p. 51) sees that

> a positive self-perception is crucial to functioning adequately and comfortably in one's surroundings. Self-worth and self-identity in the context of the environment become inseparable. . . . Psychologically, self-concept is the most vulnerable component therefore in the transac-

tions between minorities of color and majority [the health care professionals].

The sense of belonging is seen as crucial in the development of the self-concept.

The damaging effects on self-esteem for women diagnosed with HIV infection are only exacerbated by the shame and guilt they experience in knowing they might have infected their unborn child. An example of their poor self-esteem is reflected in how often HIV-infected abused women stood out due to the fact that they were missing teeth but they rarely asked for dental assistance. They did not think enough of themselves to request a referral to the dentist. Women, in general, repeatedly expressed eagerness about receiving good care for their children but were reluctant to seek care for themselves or their partners. They often expressed little concern about their health.

## *Social Stigma*

HIV diagnosis is still surrounded by discrimination on many levels. However, the social injustice experienced by minority women and their partners and children is even more intractable. Drug treatment trials appear to be more accessible to the more affluent, because they have been primarily located in medical centers better known in the middle-class communities. Complex medical information is better understood and better trusted by the middle class; social support agencies and specific communities (i.e., actors, interior designers, the fashion industry) have rallied in a positive manner to offer psychological and communal comfort to those infected.

In the poor communities inhabited by the HIV-infected women and children, this diagnosis presents only another blow to their fragile hold onto society. Women receiving methadone maintenance do not want medical staff to disclose their HIV infection status to staff at their methadone maintenance clinic for fear that they will lose the status they hold in the microcosmic community of their clinic. They recount how "news" of diagnoses spreads quickly despite attempts at confidentiality, and they do not want to be the target of gossip. They add that often they have to protect not just their right to privacy but their child's legacy. Obviously, this leaves them in a further alienated position because often the methadone clinic is their only social support network.

## Program Response

These recurring themes represented psychosocial barriers that prevented HIV-infected women and children from engaging in their health care. We employed the interdisciplinary team model that has been widely accepted as the most efficient and effective mode of delivery of health care (Cohen and Weisman 1986; Stuber 1989). The social worker is the hospital-based team member most qualified by training and orientation for the task of case coordination and development of community resources. The role of the social worker in this model is to bridge the distance between the medical center, the HIV-infected family members, and community resources. The traditional social work task of psychosocial assessment gives the interdisciplinary team a better understanding of the behavior exhibited by the family system, especially the HIV-infected mother. Additionally, partnerships were formed within the medical center, allowing a more natural flow and transition for women to receive methadone maintenance, obstetric and gynecological, and immunological management (Stuber 1989). Pediatric care with all its subspecialties including immunology needed to be offered simultaneously with the mother's and father's immunological or infectious disease health care (New York City Department of Health, AIDS Institute, 1989). Social workers offered individual, family, and support group counseling interventions as well as education and advocacy for the special needs of this population. For example, HIV-infected women were concerned about the ramifications of their illness and possible death in terms of the care and planning for dependent children. They needed help with making decisions regarding custody and wills. These considerations are difficult for poor people without access to lawyers or wealth as a legacy. They feared side effects of medications not only in terms of their health but how it would affect their ability to fulfill their parenting role.

In addition to the above-described partnerships and counseling interventions, we needed to design programs that addressed the unique issues confronted by this population. Because the creative programs developed to meet the needs of the homosexual community were not easily transferable to this population, AIDS/HIV organizations have slowly begun to develop specialized programs focusing on women and their families. Volunteer and fund-raising organizations expressed an interest in providing assistance but had no mechanisms to identify the population. Thus, relationships developed among the medical institutions and these specialized AIDS organizations, with the social worker acting as a broker in program planning. The nature of these relationships, more informal and grass roots in origin, was an asset, because this population had a distrust of formal organizations and authority based on a history of discrimination and marginal involvement with the larger society.

On the pediatric wards and specialized HIV family care clinics, programs already successful with other catastrophically ill pediatric populations were adapted for this new group. Programs such as the Clown Care Unit of the Big Apple Circus, Starlight, and the Make-A-Wish Foundation have been supportive to children and families in giving them an opportunity to experience relief from the burdensome routine of intensive medical care. Their intervention had to be modified, at times, due to some of the unique aspects of this population—for example, modifications in granting "wish trips" to Disneyland to children with AIDS coming from extended family or foster family situations. Many more relatives accompanied the child, because single parents or grand-parents, who at times spoke limited English, were unaccustomed to traveling long distances without several key family members.

Another community resource identified due to the high risk of abuse and neglect of these medically fragile and often developmentally delayed children was that of specialized preventive child welfare services. By 1988, foster care agencies were receptive to accepting HIV-infected children for placement. Many developed specialized units, which had additional staff and funding to provide a broader range of services. However, fewer child welfare agencies developed specialized preventive care programs. Through early intervention, outreach, or perinatal transmission research projects, HIV-seropositive pregnant women were identified at an increasing rate. This led to a growing pool of relatively asymptomatic women with infants at risk for infection. This cohort differed from previous cohorts that were identified as the result of the child's symptomatology and/or abandonment. These pregnant women are identified as the result of outreach and education efforts. They had better resources and kept their children at home. However, their resources were limited and they were at high risk for family disorganization once diagnosed with HIV. Under stress, some with histories of alcoholism or drug abuse returned to chemical dependency, and in some families with a history of domestic violence abuse recurred. Therefore, access to a child welfare prevention program was essential. The utility of such programs is demonstrated in the following example.

Renee was pregnant and HIV positive, but asymptomatic on enrollment in a perinatal transmission project. Her daughter was 5 years old
and HIV seronegative; she feared for her unborn child. As a single
parent, her ability to maintain her family was limited due to her history
of depression and intermittent alcoholism and intravenous-drug use.
She was bisexual but maintained no real long-term relationships. Neither father of her children was a real support to her. Her own two sisters
had very limited resources; one sister was under treatment for a severe
cardiac condition.

After delivery of her second child and the onset of her own AIDS
symptoms, Renee became increasingly anxious. She was concerned
primarily about her ability to provide for the children if she became
further disabled. She accepted a referral to a child prevention program
at a specialized HIV support program.

This mother received professional counseling at home, homemaker
service after her hospitalization, and other concrete supports. These
interventions prevented placement of her two children for almost 2 years.
After 2 years, under the stress of HIV symptomatology, she returned to
intravenous-drug and alcohol use. She made use of preventive service
interventions to have her children placed in a distant relative's home.

## Enhancing the Setting

To combat the stigma of attending an AIDS clinic, improve compliance,
and thwart isolation, we worked with pediatric AIDS fund-raising organizations and other volunteer groups to enhance our settings. Children
Immunology Research Fund, Inc., donated children's furniture. Children's Hope Foundation donated playroom toys and snacks for the waiting areas. The waiting areas were transformed from traditional municipal
hospital waiting rooms to a community center–like atmosphere. Volunteers trained by another AIDS organization, Northern Lights Alternative,
greeted patients and played with infants and children; they held infants
when parents needed to attend to their own medical care, and they
distributed snacks and charitable donations of baby food and clothing.
Families of greater means began bringing used clothes for distribution to
needier participants. Parenting tips began to be exchanged, and women
who avoided attending support groups began to speak informally about
their experiences and their symptoms. Many women remained in the
waiting area long after their medical needs were attended to. It appeared

many looked forward to their next appointment and were disappointed when they did not have to return for 6 months, if their condition was stable. They apparently took increasing pride in dressing their children for clinic appointments and would bring them dressed in special attire around the holidays. These responses were reinforced by staff, and by community visitors who developed special programs. The socialization around the clinic appointment became a powerful antidote to the stigma and isolation they experienced in the community.

## Development of Community Resources: The Religious Organization as a Paradigm

A neighborhood church in 1985 reached out to our medical center known for treating HIV-infected children. A pediatrician in the medical center was a parishioner at the local parish; she was the initial link between clergy and the medical center's pediatric AIDS social work coordinator. Although the pediatrician was not directly responsible for the care of HIV-infected children, she was aware of their needs. The initial efforts between the two organizations were around traditional Christmas gift giving; this was the beginning of a model program. The first year, the clergy made a Christmas appeal and collected funds to be given to the head nurse to buy Christmas gifts and candy. As the clergy became more aware of the needs of the children and their families, the parishioners began offering to provide more assistance. The gift giving became more personalized. The initial participation in Christmas giving expanded to all holidays. The clinic began to use holidays as a way to celebrate life, marking the passing of seasons with joy and further enhancing the appeal of the setting. Children, mothers, and eventually fathers would come to the clinic to celebrate with staff and members of the neighborhood parish, not only on Christmas but on Valentine's Day, Mother's Day, Halloween, and birthdays (of staff as well as children).

The involvement of the first parish served to inspire others who were interested in assisting HIV-infected families. One group from a neighboring state originally planned to give Christmas presents to 28 children hospitalized for infusion of intravenous gamma-globulin. This grew into 250 personally wrapped gifts, a fully decorated tree, candy, and cookies. The second parish was initially guided not by clergy but by an active parishioner; she involved her fellow choir members and other parishioners as she learned more about the children and their families. The response of her fellow parishioners led to an ongoing commitment to HIV-infected children and families not only in the neighboring state but in the following year to local children.

Key to the development of each project at the two parishes was the organizers' ability to tell more personal accounts about the children and their families. Although both efforts started as informal grass-roots projects, within a year of inception both moved into the formal structure within their organizations.

Also, both projects gave the initiator an opportunity to break down the economic and racial barriers and bias about HIV infection, especially about poor minority families with histories of drug use. The distance between the two parishes and actual contact with HIV-infected families was shortened when they proposed to "Adopt-a-Family." Each parish indicated they could "adopt" a certain number of families for the holidays, including the exchange of names and addresses, direct personal gift giving for each member of the family, and preparation of a holiday dinner, according to the cultural traditions of the family. Families who had refused public health nurses or social workers in their homes were unanimously accepting of a holiday visit from the two identified parishes. For the first time, the parishioner and clergyman met directly with infected families. This was only the beginning of an ongoing relationship that developed into a newly identified support system for previously isolated families.

The acts of charity or gift giving evolved to take on a more personal meaning for the families involved in the project. Social and emotional isolation was reduced. The women's self-image improved, and the social stigma of HIV infection was ameliorated for the women. An example of this was Renee and her two children. Renee was previously identified as having received preventive services. Renee and her two children were one of the first families enrolled in the Adopt-a-Family project.

> She requested a scooter for her 5-year-old and clothes for her newborn and, when pressed, indicated that she had always wanted a waffle iron so she could make waffles for her 5-year-old. She received these gifts for Christmas as well as other small gifts for herself, her children, and her sister, who assisted her when she could. She also received Christmas dinner.
>
> However, it was not until she was hospitalized 6 weeks later for pneumonia and had no visitors that she began to truly appreciate being

"adopted" by the local church. The social worker placed the call, with Renee's permission, to the clergyman. Visitors arrived the next day with the small necessities Renee had no access to, such as a toothbrush, a radio, and pajamas; they also brought food. These were luxuries for a woman in a municipal hospital with no phone, television, money, or access to the outside community. On discharge, they brought her a coat and stocked her empty shelves at home. For the first time in many years, Renee experienced the connection to friends who were not interested in her for sexual favors or drugs. After that she knew she had friends she could depend on.

After 2 years of sobriety, Renee returned to drug and alcohol use secondary to her anxiety about her increased HIV symptomatology. The shame and guilt of having failed her new friends kept her away for months, but in an attempt to regain her children, she returned to the clinic without an appointment asking for referral for methadone maintenance and reconnection to her old friends from the church. Contact had been maintained with the relative foster mother of the children. The clinic became the site for happy reunions between Renee, her children, and her friends. She even brought in a camera to capture pictures of all the people who made it possible for her to see her children.

The project's impact on reducing stigmatization was demonstrated also at Christmas.

A seriously ill 12-year-old child received a Christmas gift of a blue taffeta party dress. Although monitored and on intravenous medication, she managed to open the beautifully wrapped box to see her party dress. Her foster mother offered to take it home but she refused to let it go. She had never had the opportunity to have or wear such a dress and was not going to take a chance and part with it.

Families also now had allies in their fight against harassment and discrimination. This next case illustrates the role of advocacy in the face of harassment and discrimination.

Anita, a young black woman with two biological children and six kinship foster children, was "adopted" by the outreach committee and choir of one of the affiliated parishes. Anita's two sisters had died the previous year within 24 hours of each other. One sister, Liz, had a history of drug use and AIDS; she died outside a crack house on a cold December day of exposure. Anita's older sister died of cardiac arrest

24 hours later. Anita was not prepared to take on six nieces and nephews, two of whom were HIV seropositive, but she could not accept unfamiliar placement for her young family members. She kept the children between two very small apartments, one of which her sister lived in before her death.

The church volunteer offered to do more than provide food, clothing, and gifts; she offered her support and friendship in a crisis. One Saturday morning, Anita placed a call to her new friend. She was being harassed by her landlord. The landlord wanted her and the children out of her sister's apartment. She needed both apartments to house herself and the eight children; she ran up and down the flight of stairs to watch over everyone. One evening the police were called five times, arriving at her door with guns drawn on two occasions. By 10 A.M. she was frightened and exhausted. In desperation she called, hoping for solace, maybe advice and help. That Saturday morning, the volunteer called the police precinct to complain about the visits with unholstered guns and the legal aid office near Anita's home.

In the end, the landlord stopped harassing Anita, and Anita learned she could rely on her new friends from the church for support. Over the following months, the church volunteers carpeted her paint-splattered floors and provided beds for the boys. By summer the diocese and the church's outreach committee subsidized summer camp for three of the healthy boys.

The advocacy and support Anita obtained from the church volunteer sustained her in times of crisis. Both had to recognize the great disparity in their life-styles that made the relationship difficult and uncomfortable for each at times, but both valued the opportunity to know each other.

The clergyman's role evolved to provide solace even though religious affiliation had rarely been discussed. He understood the guilt and isolation experienced by family members caring for AIDS patients; he had heard grandmothers speak of self-blame or their perceptions of themselves as sinners or criminals for having HIV illness in the family. Families viewed the spiritual connection with the clergy as imparting a sense of belonging to a larger community and representing forgiveness. His presence and his parish's sponsorship of special events and projects led families to express improved feelings of self-worth and diminished emotionally debilitating despair. He represented the link between the HIV-infected community and the "respected" church community. Parish members began to express interest in becoming foster parents in the event of the death or illness of a parent they knew through the project.

# Conclusion

These programs suggest a means of diminishing the distress experienced by HIV-infected mothers and infants while allowing the general community an opportunity to express concern, compassion, and hope. As the barriers to obtaining care were diminished, engagement in health care improved. As our volunteer taught us, she cannot change the course of the illness, but she can change the "color of the sky and bring the stars back" to the darkening lives of isolated women and children.

# References

Centers for Disease Control: Telephone data from hot line information recording. Atlanta, GA, Centers for Disease Control, January 1990

Cohen MA, Weisman HW: A biopsychosocial approach to AIDS. Psychosomatics 27:245–249, 1986

Bloom M: Life Span Development. New York, Macmillan, 1980

Dokecki P, Baumeister A, Kupstas F: Biomedical and social aspects of pediatric AIDS. Journal of Early Intervention 3:99–113, 1989

Garbarino J, Sherman D: High-risk neighborhoods and high-risk families: the human ecology of child maltreatment. Child Dev 51:188–199, 1980

Germain CB, Gitterman A: The Life Model of Social Work. New York, Columbia University Press, 1980

Honey E: AIDS and the inner city: critical issues. Social Casework 69:365–370, 1988

Lewert G: Children and AIDS. Social Casework 69:348–354, 1988

New York City Department of Health: AIDS Surveillance Update. New York, New York City Department of Health, February 26, 1989

New York City Department of Health, AIDS Institute: Focus on AIDS 1:6–7, 1989

Shernoff M: Why every social worker should be challenged by AIDS. Social Work 35:5–8, 1990

Stuber ML: Coordination of care for pediatric AIDS: the development of a maternal-child HIV task force. Dev Behav Pediatr 10:201–204, 1989

*Chapter 12*

# Clinical Care of Pediatric HIV Infection: Caregiver and Institutional Issues

Penelope K.G. Krener, M.D.

*T*he first wave of acquired immunodeficiency syndrome (AIDS) in the United States engulfed homosexual men and recipients of transfusions and blood products. The human immunodeficiency virus (HIV) epidemic is nearing the end of its first decade, and it is already clear that it will cut short a generation of young homosexual men, of families with hemophilia, and of intravenous-drug users and their children. The second wave of the infection is sweeping over a younger population of intravenous-drug users, their children, and those to whom the virus is spread venereally (Department of Health and Human Services 1986). A first generation of care providers are also beginning to be lost, either because they themselves are ill or seropositive, or through exhaustion and burnout. Responses to the HIV epidemic must be devised while the health care system itself is in transformation. Those who have always taken care of children—parents, teachers, pediatricians, family practitioners, and child psychiatrists—must now learn how to take care of children who have AIDS.

The spread of HIV is a medical epidemic and also a social one. The care provider for patients infected with HIV operates in several dimensions of the epidemic (AIDS Surveillance Unit 1989; Belfer et al. 1988). One dimension is that of the progression of HIV infection within the individual, as a chronic illness eventuating in death. Another dimension is the psychosocial context of the individual person with AIDS. Caring

Thanks are given to Elizabeth Harrison, M.D., for sharing materials from the Sacramento AIDS Foundation Hand-to-Hand training manual and for organizing the group of volunteers working with children and families with HIV infection.

for a person infected with HIV, especially as an outpatient, requires understanding of the following aspects of the patient's life: What is the person's cultural context and how is illness dealt with in that culture? Is the family intact? Is the family functional, or are family members ill or addicted? Is there an underlying illness such as hemophilia? Does the patient have a mental illness or substance abuse disorder as well as HIV infection? How poor or socially isolated is the patient? The psychiatrist must consider the patient's psychiatric status (Does the patient meet criteria for a DSM-III-R [American Psychiatric Association 1987] diagnosis?), his or her cultural context (e.g., minority status), socioeconomic level, family interactions, and function, and whether there is an underlying medical illness. The child psychiatrist considers all of these, but also the young patient's stage of development. Over the course of a lengthy illness, the individual patient continues to grow as a person. Young adult patients whose lives are cut short by a terminal illness compress into the truncated span an intense culmination and attempt to resolve and complete their relationships and creations. Children achieve developmental milestones, acquire new knowledge before they die of AIDS, and become unforgettable parts of the lives of those who take care of them. Unable to accurately guess how long a child with HIV infection will live, the caregiver must devise approaches that combine good medicine with good nurturing, making care decisions that allow the best possible normal opportunities for the child.

## Care of Children and Adolescents Infected With HIV

The diagnosis of HIV infection in the infant, whether or not accompanied by a diagnosis in the mother, devastates the family. Psychological support is urgently needed at this point and ideally should be incorporated into the ongoing medical management along with monitoring of growth, nutrition, interaction with caregivers, and developmental progression or plateauing. When neurological involvement develops, it is necessary to provide a stable interpersonal environment with consistent caregivers (Krener 1987). In outpatient management of children with HIV infection, it is important to remember that different family members may be at different stages in the painful process of acculturation to chronic illness and may be coping in various ways.

The infected child may also be an orphan, or a functional orphan if the parents are severely ill or addicted. However, families of children with HIV infection are often ill themselves. The adult family member with HIV disease may require the care of a parallel group of specialists, as well as needing assistance with psychosocial problems resulting from drug use or poverty, necessitating a double round of medical evaluations and follow-up visits. If infants outlive their parents, decisions about placement in public or foster care must be made, which are difficult for any child but especially so for children who are ill or neurologically compromised. However, more than one-half of newborns testing seropositive will not go on to develop HIV because seropositivity reflects maternal infection. They need a normal family environment to avoid developmental problems resulting from early isolation, abandonment, and stigmatization.

## Public Health, Outpatient Care, and Outreach

The HIV epidemic has thrown into somber prominence the aspects of the health care system that have functioned poorly to provide equal access to health care. The populations most vulnerable to HIV infection through intravenous-drug use are those who have the least basic medical care. To develop the clinical and outreach treatment programs needed to carry out preventive intervention once high-risk infants and families are identified, active advocacy is needed. Proficiency in the tactics of accessing social security, Medicaid, health services, legal counsel, and mental health resources is a necessity. Services must be differentiated to include the needs of young patients at different developmental stages. For infants, the support of their parents offers them prevention against insufficient nurturing or out-of-home placement. For school-age children, issues of discrimination and health maintenance are important. In the adolescent population, overlapping risk categories exist—psychiatric symptoms, emerging homosexuality, drug use, runaway status—and are often responded to with fragmented services. Families may experience financial and social depletion as several family members may be infected. Training in counseling, grieving, and active-listening skills is required to provide psychological support, but an interest in and concern about the patient is needed to be able to offer friendship along with clinical expertise. Volunteers and public health services may be recruited to assist with practical needs, such as providing cooking, shopping, cleaning, transportation, babysitting, respite care, and personal services to the homebound patient and family. Additional burdens fall on the health care worker as families may be isolated, alienated, and lacking support from the rest of their community, or be rejected and discriminated against. Exacting documentation of medical services to satisfy utilization review, particularly for unreimbursed patients, adds to the care provider's burden.

Community volunteer projects such as Shanti in San Francisco, Gay Men's Health Crisis in New York, and Hand-to-Hand in Sacramento have developed models to supplement the services of medical and social service workers. In Hand-to-Hand, volunteers provide service in three main areas: advocacy, practical support, and emotional support. After being recruited by media or word of mouth, they are screened in written and personal interviews. Their training includes medical overviews, experiential exercises, role-playing, acquiring specific attendant care skills, contact with panels of people with AIDS, and discussing relevant cultural issues. Volunteers are matched one to one with people with HIV disease and provide 3–6 hours a week of service for an extended time in an ongoing relationship. Often their attachment to their clients, and their response to the client's health decline, is such that they give much more time than expected. Weekly or biweekly group support and supervision of volunteers are usually provided, with phone and emergency backup for medical and mental health consultation or for emotional support.

## The Pediatric Specialty Clinic

Some infants with congenital HIV infection deteriorate and die within months, but many youngsters infected perinatally with HIV are not diagnosed until early childhood and live with HIV as a chronic illness into their school years. The necessity for hospitalizations can be reduced if children receive regular clinic care, preferably in a clinic staffed by a multidisciplinary team and geared to treating children with HIV infection. Pediatric care should be comprehensive and aimed at secondary prevention. Treatment includes monitoring growth, development, and nutrition, administering gamma-globulin or antiviral agents, and treating intercurrent adventitious infections. Because several subspecialists, including pediatric infectious disease specialists, neurologists, and nutritionists, must cooperate for adequate maintenance of the child's HIV infection, the HIV clinic must do much more liaison than is common for specialty clinics or have an internal structure that facilitates multidisciplinary care. A pediatric nurse specialist can help to integrate the information into a practical treatment program, and a social worker is a vital member of the team because the social problems underlying vulnerability to HIV and those resulting from it are so extensive.

The model clinic is one equipped to provide integrated and coordinated services for pediatric, teen, obstetrics and gynecology, and family practice care. A full-time clinic coordinator to schedule clinic visits and maintain contact between patients and community agencies and clinic staff will maximize continuity and follow-up. This avoids the fragmentation of services that occurs when families must attend different clinics for contraception, infectious disease treatment, and general medical care. It improves record keeping, reduces missed appointments, and promotes confidentiality. The clinic care team should meet regularly to discuss clinic protocols and patient care issues and to update team members on patients' status. Ideally, women will be provided with care similar to that for children for health maintenance and treatment of acute illness and infection. Also, they could gain information about contraceptive alternatives and how to assert to partners their need for safe sexual practices. Anticipatory guidance about their child's development will be most useful in the context of the child's chronic condition, as is planning for conservatorship status or wills and recruitment of supportive family members and friends as parents become ill and less able to care for their children.

Outpatient issues in caring for the child with HIV infection go beyond the usual problems of chronic illness, growth, nutrition, and well-being because of the child's vulnerability to infections and to discrimination, even in a situation where the school is accepting (Price 1986; Rubenstein 1986). The American Academy of Pediatrics has taken the position that children with AIDS should attend school unless they cannot handle their secretions, they bite other children, or they have open skin sores (American Academy of Pediatrics Committee on Infectious Diseases 1986; Black 1986; Centers for Disease Control 1988). However, immunodeficient children should be protected as much as possible from contagious illnesses in the school population. The pediatrician and child psychiatrist will be asked to make more decisions about school field trips, overnight visits with friends, and special occasions that may pose special risks, but that are important to the child having as normal a childhood experience as possible. Because AIDS is not only a new chronic illness that requires much education, but also one that is stigmatized, the physician may be called on in special ways to advocate for the child if there are discriminatory obstacles to participating in school or community activities. For adolescents, social issues such as sexual abuse or drug behaviors must be addressed along with medical issues.

The tactical and emotional problems posed by an illness that may affect several members of a family are added to by the extensive social problems of families who may have been dysfunctional or involved with drugs before developing HIV. Supporting the child's family requires assessment of possible parental dysfunction due to multiple risk factors, including substance abuse or chaotic life situations, which can be a difficult task in pediatric settings. The impact of the diagnosis is powerful; psychiatric symptomatology is prevalent in persons who have recently learned that they are seropositive. Each member of the family, including the child patient, must pass through successive stages of coming to terms with the reality that one or more of them has an incurable illness. The team caring for the child with HIV infection may find it hard to allow time for this process to occur, especially if they feel that opportunities for prevention are being missed. They may see the family's resistance as frank medical noncompliance. Most difficult are the situations in which a family member responsible for carrying out the care plan is thought to have a subtle psychiatric condition or an organic mental disorder related to AIDS dementia complex (ADC) or substance abuse.

Evaluation by a psychiatrist can assist in defining the family's strengths and weaknesses. Psychiatric advocacy can specifically address the clinical need for orchestrated care in order to optimize the child's development and minimize erosion of morale and skills. The child psychiatrist's specific skills are needed for diagnostic differentiation between neurological, psychiatric, and environmental causes of developmental failure, but only by becoming a part of the outpatient team over time can the child psychiatrist best plot the trajectory of the child's emotional development.

## The Hospital Ward

When children with HIV infection come into the hospital, their stays are often longer than the other patients on the pediatric service, their recovery from infections is slower, and they experience more complications. Their families may visit infrequently because they are ill themselves, or because they are dysfunctional, or because of inability to manage the expense of travel to the hospital. If the child forms attachments to other children in the hospital whose families are more functional, their own deprivation is felt more intensely by them and by the staff caring for them. Nursing staff often must find the emotional energy to comfort the angry or sad child who believed that the day of discharge had come, only to be told that discharge is postponed because of a relapse or complication. The child may not be able to understand or accept the contingencies for discharge and may see the delay in going home as a broken promise. Nursing and medical staff may have to find ways to explain the complex and intersecting reasons for making a medical decision about readiness for discharge to a child who has not achieved formal operations–level information processing.

The child with HIV infection who comes into the hospital may need psychiatric consultation to help evaluate depression, ADC, or the functioning of his or her family. Inserting himself or herself into a series of consultants all visiting the child, the psychiatrist must find ways to understand and communicate how the particular child is coping with the illness. Some children withdraw, to conserve their emotional energy and to discourage well-meaning professionals from engaging them in confusing encounters that may not lead to attachments.

This may present a picture similar to depression. Others have learned to capitalize on being "special" by virtue of their HIV infection and hold court in bed, waiting for attention. To understand where the child is in his or her cycle of adaptation to the illness and in the process of comprehending its implications requires not only spending time with the child, but also getting to know the family directly or learning about them through those who know the child and family.

Consultation-liaison skills are essential for operating in a multidisciplinary field. Psychiatric consultants must be prepared to help caregivers of children with HIV infection deal with fear, contempt, grief, and burnout—four feeling patterns not usually encountered in pediatrics. The ordinary healthy denial of death is more difficult in the case of HIV infection, an illness that is largely invisible and that kills young patients. Fear of contagion overwhelms factual information. Most medical services dealing with AIDS patients progressively overcome this fear (Kreiner 1987), but each psychiatric consultant must be prepared to sensitively assess the stage of understanding of the service to which he or she consults. Feelings of contempt for families whose behavior they blame for the child's illness may be difficult for medical and mental health personnel to acknowledge, especially as they may coexist with unacceptable but real racial attitudes and personal convictions about sexual practices or drug abuse. Psychiatric consultation may help to neutralize negative feelings interfering with care, by identifying difficult feelings and by showing that the infected parent is also a victim. Pediatricians and obstetricians may be more vulnerable to personal grief when their young patients die than those in specialties serving older patients (Sack et al. 1984). Their colleagues must support them in managing that grief.

Burnout, the well-described configuration of exhaustion, depersonalization, and feelings of failure, occurs frequently among those who care for patients with HIV infection. Professional exhaustion and successive losses without a recovery period may make it difficult for those who care for AIDS patients to properly care for themselves. Support from psychiatric colleagues can help clinicians' adaptation to struggle with their patients' illness over the long haul.

## Psychiatric Inpatient Care

Psychiatric units will admit increasing numbers of youth with HIV infection. Increasingly, child psychiatrists will need to become proficient at neuropsychiatric assessment and management of medical psychiatric situations. Staff fear of contagion or tendency to avoid attachment to a person with a terminal illness may become obstacles to care unless special training and support are offered to health care providers. ADC and depression may prolong psychiatric hospitalizations, but third-party carriers may deny reimbursement, placing adolescent inpatient units in a familiar conflict between program needs and patient needs.

The American Academy of Child and Adolescent Psychiatry (1989) has developed a guideline summary on specific inpatient issues. It states that HIV status should not be mandatorily assessed before admission and is not a reason to deny admission as long as the patient can comply with infection-control measures, does not have aggressive sexual or biting behavior, and has access to medical support. Universal precautions procedures are now standard in hospitals. Containment of risk-producing behaviors is possible in well-staffed settings, so needed psychiatric admissions can be offered even to behaviorally unstable patients if the acuity of their staffing need is identified.

Psychiatric inpatient stays offer an opportunity for thorough assessment of developmental, neuropsychiatric, and affective effects on the patient. Because AIDS is a life-threatening sexually transmitted disease, child and adolescent psychiatrists must routinely take thorough sexual histories. Evaluation of families must include determining whether other family members are also ill, and whether they have the energy and resources necessary to support an adolescent with possible health problems after his or her discharge. Patients with HIV spectrum disease present difficult problems in all diagnostic areas; DSM-III-R Axis I diagnoses may include developmental, organic, affective, substance abuse, and adjustment disorders. Axis II diagnoses are common, in part produced by deprivation resulting from drug abuse, genetic factors, exposure to prenatal toxins, or child abuse associated with drug use. Axis III diagnoses are frequent as the illness progresses. Axis IV levels of psychosocial stress are typically high, and Axis V global assessment of functioning (highest level of adaptive functioning in the past year) may fluctuate widely within a year's time.

Treatment of substance-abusing youth and those who also have another Axis I disorder always poses management challenges, but when such youngsters are HIV positive, the stakes are higher because of pressure for education to prevent the spread of the virus. Adolescents must be questioned carefully about risk behaviors, which may include shared use of sharp implements for cutting (DiClemente, in press). Adolescents with psychiatric symptoms are no less sexually active than their peers. Homosexual adolescents may evince psychiatric symptoms as a result of the pressures they experience about their homosexuality (Remafedi 1987) before they disclose their sexual orientation. They must be helped to feel that the psychiatric staff is nonjudgmental and willing to work with them to discover ways to live safely as they feel they need to. Careful evaluation of the youngster's emotional state and cognitive capacity should precede communication of difficult instructions, which includes communicating antibody test results, because they may be unable to incorporate important information or to control their emotional reactions. Knowledge alone is not enough for behavior change, and psychiatric hospitalizations are opportunities for exploring attitudes and coping styles that may interfere with youngsters' connecting knowledge to their own life after discharge. Group sessions may be used for role-playing and other exercises to help youth practice the assertiveness and social skills they will need to implement self-protective behavior.

Decisions about testing for and disclosure of seropositivity may need to be made during the psychiatric stay. Regardless of results of testing, this vulnerable population should be educated about high-risk behavior. Planning what information to give children and adolescents, who should give it, and how it should be framed must be done with reference to cognitive development, the family's stage of disclosure in their community, and the youngster's relationship with the medical caregiver. Sharing of HIV status should be in compliance with state and federal law and should protect both the patient's confidentiality and health care options.

# Caregiver Issues in the Care of HIV Spectrum Disease

## *Communication Among Care Providers*

Children affected by HIV infection are exposed not only through medical events such as transfusion, but also through social ailments such as intravenous-drug abuse. Therefore, those who care for them must be skilled in more than medical care. For the child to live with a chronic illness, physicians must work with the family, which may be ailing or dysfunctional. It is necessary to coordinate with the child's school to protect the child from discrimination and avoidable infection. If substance abuse is ongoing in the child's family, the physician may need to seek the intervention of social agencies. No single caregiver can possess all the skills or energy that are needed to care for a child with AIDS. Working in a multidisciplinary team bolsters individual clinicians and ensures against feeling unable to respond alone to all the needs of the patient.

Volunteers may have allied themselves with the child and family. If they are invited to help with the child's care by bringing the child to the clinic or visiting in the hospital, the familiar division of professional and nonprofessional roles may be disrupted. Nurses and parents may need the volunteer to help sustain the child through procedures and hospital separations, but volunteers cannot officially read medical charts and must depend on medical personnel to communicate medical information, so they can support and prepare the child. For some pediatricians and pediatric nurses, depending on an individual without medical training to support them and their patient may be experienced as a departure from their comfortable professional expectation of mastery and competence.

There is much to be learned by professionals about the experience of illness from those without the bias of medical training.

Placement in group homes and institutional settings is often resorted to for AIDS orphans, but diluted parenting and exposure to a larger number of children in their living setting may compromise secondary prevention of complications of HIV positivity for small children. New programs for caring for infants orphaned by AIDS are needed, particularly in areas with high prevalence of AIDS infection in children. At a time when public funding is scarce, it is urgently necessary to develop new, integrated health care systems and programs to place boarder babies and to increase subsidized medical foster homes. Professional advocacy should be added to local pressures to make such programs possible.

CDC recommends against group settings for HIV-infected children younger than age 3 years because they are highly vulnerable to opportunistic infections. Parenting is spread thinner in group homes. Group home care is often costlier than family care with associated support services. Psychiatrists may help in the task of recruiting and maintaining foster families advocating for children who have lost their birth families. They can assist with evaluations that encourage certification of relatives as foster parents, entitled to the same payments and support as other foster parents, to enlarge the pool. They can support foster parents who may face criticism from and rejection by friends and relatives for bringing a child with AIDS into their home to raise with their own children. Families need guidance to know how to explain the illness and death of the foster child to their own children and to their children's friends. Such opportunities for secondary prevention of the psychological toll of AIDS in children through psychological support for extended families and foster families will reduce the number of psychiatric casualties to which we will respond in the future. Reimbursement modes for such powerful augmenters of psychiatric skill are inadequate, and this fact should be challenged by psychiatrists motivated to do this work.

## Constraints of Existing Service Systems

AIDS, a chronic illness posing formidable requirements for management, has disproportionately afflicted a population whose previous health care utilization patterns were no better than the service delivery systems available to them. The present health care system is a mosaic of public funding, private insurance, and self-payment, which has many missing pieces. Deficiencies in preventive health care services for poor and minority patients, including the lack of drug treatment programs, are part of the reason why AIDS has spread more rapidly among the medically and socially disenfranchised in this country (Mays and Cochran 1987). The existing system has been unable to meet the needs of the larger numbers of persons with HIV infection in poor areas (Report of the Presidential Commission on the Human Immunodeficiency Virus Epidemic 1988). Minority populations at risk must be targeted for medical, obstetric, nutritional, and mental health services and for drug treatment, education, and counseling. Low-income families with multiple medical problems must travel to different sites for care: to methadone maintenance clinics, Medicaid agencies, prenatal clinics, pediatric clinics, and welfare offices. Referrals may be difficult to implement and follow-up may be limited.

Models do exist for the kind of program needed for children with HIV spectrum disease. Culturally sensitive, federally sponsored, comprehensive care systems, such as the National Cancer Institute's Pediatric Oncology Program and the Developmental Disabilities Program supported by the Offices of Human Development Services and of Maternal and Child Health, are examples. Child psychiatrists should become part of such model programs for AIDS and should advocate for their replications in local communities. Public Law 99-457 establishes a program to provide early intervention services to handicapped or developmentally delayed infants and toddlers (0–24 months) to begin in the school year 1990–1991. Children whose developmental delay is caused by AIDS should be eligible for such services, but they will require advocacy and referral in order to access them.

Statutes for protection of the rights and safety of children, although variable from state to state, have all required reexamination in the face of the AIDS epidemic. If the parents are dead and other relatives are uninvolved, the state has full responsibility for the child, but if a parent has voluntarily placed the child in foster care, then the parent retains the right of approval. If the state has legal responsibility for the child, it may seek parental approval before making any decision involving the child. Children who are wards of the state may have no one to sign to authorize their participation in experimental or innovative investigational treatment programs, so they cannot receive optimum care that might alleviate their symptoms, reduce complicating illnesses, and improve their quality of life.

## Transference and Countertransference Issues

The statistics outlined in the introduction make it clear that racial and cultural awareness must be part of the medical response to the AIDS epidemic. Attitudes about race and class are deep, often preaware patterns of simplifying information about people. Health care providers and mental health workers who have not grown up in poverty, who have not been targets of violence, and who have not been discriminated against must listen carefully to their patients who have. Otherwise, they may not realize that recommendations that have logical coherence from a public health point of view may be interpreted as inappropriate or even genocidal from a social point of view.

An example is the response of some members of the black community in New York City to a proposed needle-exchange program to prevent the spread of AIDS (Dalton 1989). Some leaders who had struggled unsuccessfully and with insufficient support from local government to eradicate the drug epidemic in their communities felt that this was an example of a solution authored by whites that did not take into account the entire social problem—more minority youth are killed each year from use of drugs and the violence surrounding them than die of AIDS. A long experience of feeling dictated or condescended to, of having programs imposed from outside the community, and of not being heard about the needs of their communities may make minority patients hesitant to form alliances with the physicians who now are trying to treat HIV spectrum disease.

Countertransference is powerful for the health care worker or volunteer who is HIV infected, or who is a recovered drug addict, is homosexual, or has hemophilia. Identification with the ill person, or loyalty to a shared group, makes them ready to involve themselves in the intense physical and emotional care required. Health care providers may be HIV positive but fear discovery, malpractice claims, loss of occupation, and choice of other providers by their patients, at a time when they feel indispensable to their work. Mental health providers may experience identification anxiety and depression (Simmons-Alling 1984; Wolcott et al. 1985). Successive losses of patients and colleagues with insufficient time to grieve between bereavements, and the attrition of friends and support systems, drain the spirit of this special group who can be uniquely effective caregivers. The child psychiatrist can offer individual and group psychotherapy services to other outreach workers and to volunteers, even if he or she is limited by time or reimbursement modes from caring for many AIDS patients directly.

Support for such groups should have five goals:

1. Creating working relationships with a shared purpose and ready support (Beardslee and De Maso 1982)
2. Supporting activity rather than passivity, but accepting limitations and being willing to change goals and approaches over time to help avoid discouragement as the patient loses ground
3. Allowing time to grieve and recover after a patient dies
4. Avoiding inadequate rest, respite, and restoration
5. Taking pride in special care and attentiveness for patients and avoiding self-criticism for not being able to accomplish the impossible

Group and individual therapeutic support is vital to protect committed care providers whose personal involvement with the epidemic may make them feel that there are no outs, not even burnout. These providers may chose to live under pressures that may make them more vulnerable and, without support, potentially less able to help their clients.

## Conclusion

Child psychiatrists will increasingly be asked to consult to clinicians and to community programs whose clients are infected with HIV (Krener and Miller 1989). They may be asked to assess parenting skills in the high-risk mother-infant pair at the time of delivery. Techniques of evaluating mother-infant bonding and infant neurological maturity and modulation may assist in identifying infants who will be difficult to parent or mothers who have limited parenting skills. Child psychiatrists are well equipped to evaluate the causes of developmental compromise—neurological, illness related, or environmental—and to recommend remedial plans. They are trained to hear the quiet or nonverbal voices that the child may use to express secret fears or idiosyncratic understandings and to back-translate family innuendo into open formulations allowing for change. They are able to understand the cognitive and emotional riptides within the adolescent, whose rising intellectual capacity, stormy sexuality, and need for differentiation from the family may wash onto difficult social shoals of drug abuse or environmental disorganization. However, the usual training of child psychiatrists does not inure them to untimely death, provide them with formulas for helping clients deal with poverty and violence, or give them more than a pidgin vocabulary to converse in unfamiliar meanings systems of different subcultures. Training in various therapeutic modalities will insulate them little from the erosive losses of caring for dying young people (Adams-Greenly and Moynihan 1983; Furman 1974; Gardner 1985; Horstman and McKusisk 1986). Their insights into their own countertransference vulnerabilities offer limited protection from the professional self-doubts stirred by serving disenfranchised, addicted, or bereaved clients who are overwhelmed and for whom the consultant cannot command auxiliary services. Therefore, they must learn, with and from their patients, ways to deepen their skills to respond to the AIDS epidemic and to the underlying social problems that have hastened its spread among young parents and children.

# References

Adams-Greenly M, Moynihan RT: Helping the children of fatally ill parents. Am J Orthopsychiatry 53:219–229, 1983

AIDS Surveillance Unit: AIDS Surveillance Unit update. New York, New York City Department of Health, March 29, 1989

American Academy of Child and Adolescent Psychiatry: Policy statement: AIDS and Psychiatric Hospitalization of Children and Adolescents. Washington, DC, American Academy of Child and Adolescent Psychiatry, 1989

American Academy of Pediatrics Committee on Infectious Diseases: School attendance of children and adolescents with human T lymphotrophic virus III/lymphadenopathy-associated virus infection. Pediatrics 77:430–432, 1986

Beardslee WR, De Maso DR: Staff groups in a pediatric hospital: content and coping. Am J Orthopsychiatry 52:712–718, 1982

Belfer ML, Krener PK, Miller FB: AIDS in children and adolescents. J Am Acad Child Adolesc Psychiatry 27:147–151, 1988

Black JL: AIDS: preschool and school issues. J Sch Health 56:93–95, 1986

Centers for Disease Control: Guidelines for effective school health education to prevent the spread of AIDS. MMWR 37:717–721, 1988

Dalton HL: AIDS in blackface. Daedalus 118:205–227, 1989

Department of Health and Human Services: An Occasional Report on Runaway and Homeless Youth Data. Office of Human Development Services. Data on youth identified as "Possibly Suicidal." Washington, DC, U.S. Government Printing Office, 1986, pp 1–7

DiClemente RJ, Ponton LE, Hartley D, et al: Prevalence of HIV-related high-risk sexual and drug-related behaviors among adolescents with severe emotional disturbances: preliminary results, in Troubled Adolescents and HIV Infection: Issues in Prevention and Treatment. Edited by Woodruff JO, Doherty D, Garrison-Athey J. Washington, DC, Georgetown University, CASSP Technical Assistance Center (in press)

Furman E: A Child's Parent Dies: Studies in Childhood Bereavement. New Haven, CT, Yale University Press, 1974

Gardner GG: The dying child and adolescent—ethical perspectives, in Understanding Human Behavior in Health and Illness. Edited by Simons RC. Baltimore, MD, Williams & Wilkins, 1985, pp 299–302

Horstman W, McKusisk L: The impact of AIDS on the physician, in What to Do About AIDS. Edited by McKusisk L. San Francisco, University of California Press, 1986

Krener PG: Impact of the diagnosis of AIDS on hospital care of an infant. Clin Pediatr 26:93–97, 1987

Krener PG, Miller FB: Psychiatric response to HIV spectrum disease in children and adolescents. J Am Acad Child Adolesc Psychiatry 28:596–605, 1989

Mays VM, Cochran SD: Acquired immune deficiency syndrome and black Americans: special psychosocial issues. Public Health Rep 102:224–231, 1987

Price JH: AIDS, the schools, and policy issues. J Sch Health 56:137–140, 1986

Remafedi G: Adolescent homosexuality: psychosocial and medical implications. Pediatrics 79:331–337, 1987

Report of the Presidential Commission on the Human Immunodeficiency Virus Epidemic. Washington, DC, U.S. Government Printing Office, June 1988

Rubenstein A: Schooling for children with acquired immune deficiency syndrome. J Pediatr 109:242–244, 1986

Sack W, Fritz G, Krener PG, et al: Death and the pediatric house officer revisited. Pediatrics 73:676–681, 1984

Simmons-Alling S: AIDS: Psychosocial needs of the health care worker. Topics in Clinical Nursing 6:31–37, 1984

Wolcott DL, Fawzy F, Pasnau RO: Acquired immune deficiency syndrome (AIDS) and consultation liaison psychiatry. Gen Hosp Psychiatry 7:280–293, 1985

*Chapter 13*

# Psychotherapy Issues
# in Pediatric HIV and AIDS

Margaret L. Stuber, M.D.

As recently as a decade ago it was widely believed that infectious
disease was no longer much of a threat to the developed world . . .
that confidence was shattered in the early 1980s by the advent of
AIDS. (Gallo and Montagnier 1988, p. 41)

Since it first came to public awareness, the human immunodeficiency
virus (HIV) has been uniquely effective in mobilizing numerous deep-
seated irrational fears and biases, intensifying divisions of ethnicity, race,
socioeconomic status, and sexual preference. These fears and biases,
under the guise of self-protection and public safety, have resulted in
legislative action, protest marches, arson, and assault as well as family
civil wars, personnel action, and insurance rulings. Psychotherapists are
in a position to bring insight, if not reason, to this tangle of conflict and
self-destructive behavior. As the impact of acquired immunodeficiency
syndrome (AIDS) reaches to touch more and more Americans, it increasingly becomes an issue for mental health professionals.

In this chapter, I examine two particularly difficult situations encountered by psychotherapists working with children, adolescents, or
families: 1) psychotherapy with an HIV-infected child, and 2) consultation or psychotherapy with multiply infected families. Practical suggestions about how to approach specific issues raised within a therapeutic
relationship will be discussed. Because earlier chapters in this volume

This work was supported in part by Clinical Oncology Career Development Award 89-192
from the American Cancer Society.

address issues of race, ethnicity, socioeconomic status, and the particular problems of adolescents and children with hemophilia, these will not be repeated. The objective of this chapter is to assist the experienced clinician to apply his or her skills to the unique problems raised by this new virus, and by our society's response.

## The HIV-Infected Child

AIDS has replaced cancer as the disease too horrible to name (Sontag 1989). The fear and stigma of cancer have been reduced by increasing knowledge and efficacy of treatment. It is now generally accepted that it is better for children with cancer to be told their diagnosis (Slavin et al. 1982). Detailed explanations are presented to their teachers and classmates, with the understanding that this facilitates psychosocial adjustment of all concerned (Katz and Ingle-Nelson 1989).

This is not true of pediatric AIDS. Not only is the diagnosis kept secret from teachers and classmates, but parents commonly choose not to tell young infected children, fearful that they will be unable to keep the secret, and eager to shield them from societal response. Children may be told they have an unspecified blood disease or pneumonia, or even leukemia. Teachers and classmates are told only enough to protect the immunosuppressed child from exposure to contagious disease such as chicken pox, or to excuse him or her for clinic appointments. Medical personnel often will encourage parents to withhold the truth, hoping to avoid social stigma, rejection, or even overt attacks (Belfer et al. 1988; Kermani 1988).

This approach worked moderately well in the early 1980s. Few children were infected, and most died relatively rapidly. However, as HIV infection has become a chronic (albeit still fatal) disease in children, we must reconsider such attempts at "protection." The child who is shielded from knowledge about his or her own disease may avoid societal stigma and isolation, but at the cost of isolation within the family. Children are excellent observers, especially of their parents. When parental tension and distress are apparent, and yet poorly explained, the child will generate a number of questions. Without satisfactory answers, the child will invent his or her own answer, generally involving self-blame, punishment, and isolation. Although it may be difficult for the child to imagine something much more terrible than the reality of AIDS, the isolation and guilt that secrecy creates interfere with the child's ability to get support at a critical time. Open communication allows clarification of misinterpretations, as well as reassurance that the child will not be abandoned and that the illness is not his or her fault. We must also be aware that the child's concerns may be quite different from our own and must listen carefully. For example, an HIV-infected 7-year-old girl asked if she could give her virus to someone else. A family meeting was called by the psychotherapist to discuss the infectious nature of her illness. However, closer listening to the question revealed that the girl simply wanted to know if it was possible to get rid of the annoying intruder by giving it to a (presumably disliked) peer.

In addition to these problems of children's interpretations of events is a more pragmatic problem. It is extremely difficult to maintain a secret from children. Eventually someone slips. The child overhears a supposed private conversation, or reads an overlooked chart, or is simply told by tired or distracted medical staff. These revelations can be devastating to the child, as they simultaneously present the child with two major issues: 1) a frightening and confusing diagnosis, and 2) evidence that his or her parents and doctors have been lying. The latter fact makes the former much more difficult to address. Overcoming the resulting suspicion and betrayal can be a major, and painful, therapeutic endeavor.

Unfortunately, the solution is not as simple as saying that all secrecy should be avoided, in the interest of trust and open communication. In some, if not all, segments of American society, the irrational fear of AIDS is sufficient to motivate people to cruel and even violent behavior. (See Chapter 8, this volume, for examples.) Under such circumstances, selectivity in disclosure may appear prudent, until society's views soften. The basic flaw in this argument is that the most effective way to combat these assumptions is repeated public evidence that these children are not dangerous. Ryan White's very public struggle helped educate many people—but at great personal cost to Ryan and his family. Not all children and families are willing to be pioneers in this way. Those who can and will deserve our support. They are preparing the way for the future. Those who choose to remain private at present need our counsel as to how best to do this.

An approach that has proved workable for families with children preschool to early elementary school age is to explain the illness at a developmentally appropriate level, but without using the terms "HIV" or "AIDS." The child or family can give their own name to the "bug" that is making the child ill. Preschool-age children rarely need or understand more than very basic information about a germ or problem in the blood that makes it easier to get sick than most people. As children become more cognitively sophisticated, the amount of detail needed and understood increases.

There are a number of advantages to this approach. The child is given an explanation for the events that are happening and can ask answerable questions. Open communication is facilitated, allowing all parties to be overt about feelings and treatment. It is also a significant asset for the therapist working with the child and family. There is a name (albeit the family's or child's unique name) for the problem, and it can therefore be addressed.

At some point, however, the child must be told the full story. If at all possible this should be timed to precede the child's discovery or realization of the common name of the "bug," for the reasons discussed above. The child's exact chronologic age when he or she should be told will vary, according to the circumstances and the child's curiosity and intelligence. In most cases, however, children will figure out their diagnosis during the curious early elementary school years. Because by then it is also possible for most children to understand why the family does not want the diagnosis shared publicly, it is appropriate to talk with the child at around that age, or earlier for particularly mature children. In some cases, when HIV-induced or other developmental disabilities have impaired the child's cognitive level and impulse control, a much later age may be appropriate.

There are a number of books and videos that can be used to assist parents in discussing HIV and AIDS with young children. A bibliography of some useful resources appears at the end of this chapter. Although the child may have few questions at first, it is essential that provisions be made to answer questions as they come up. This may be complicated if there are other, particularly younger, children at home, who have not been informed about the diagnosis. Specific settings can be designated for discussions about HIV. Parents should be prepared to answer the same questions multiple times, as the child struggles to assimilate the information. A major emphasis should be dispelling common myths that the child or family members have encountered.

If the parents find the initial discussion or later talks too stressful by themselves, meetings can be held with the psychotherapist supporting the parents as they present the information. Other medical personnel may sometimes be included, if specific technical questions must be addressed, or major decisions made (such as starting or discontinuing an experimental treatment).

Parents should also be prepared for one of the most common, and earliest, questions to be asked: "Am I gonna die?" As Erma Bombeck was told by children with cancer when she was writing her most recent book, *I Want to Grow Hair, I Want to Grow Up, I Want to Go to Boise* (1989), "The first chapter should be 'Am I gonna die?' because that's what everyone thinks about when they're first diagnosed." This question is undoubtedly second only to fear of societal response as a motivation for both parents and physicians to keep the diagnosis from children. It is difficult to tolerate answering this question when the best honest answer is "not right now." As improved treatment permits more optimism, it should become somewhat easier to be honest with infected children, as it has been with children who have cancer.

Unfortunately, for the present, the issue of death is a very real part of psychotherapy with infected children. Although helping a child face death may be the most difficult task a mental health professional can undertake, it can also be among the most deeply moving. Therapist and child are forced to struggle together to face unanswerable questions: "What's it like after you die?" "Will I ever see my parents again?" "Why did this happen to me?" Studies done with children with other chronic and/or fatal diseases have demonstrated that children as young as age 6 appear to grasp the significance of their medical situation (Share 1972; Spinetta 1974). The courage children display, as well as their ability to use honesty and support, sustains the therapist who chooses to undertake this demanding and painful job.

Sensitive, open communication is the essential component of effective work with a terminally ill child. This does not mean that the therapist must repeatedly bring up or discuss the child's illness or future. Rather, there must be the clear message that *all* topics are available for discussion. For example, an 8-year-old boy reported a dream in which he was a tree being cut down while still alive. Although he was not ready to talk about the possibility of his own death, the dream allowed discussion of his thoughts about an afterlife, as well as demonstrating that his worst fears could be spoken, at least in symbolic form, and tolerated by his mother and therapist.

Similarly, the question "Why me?," although ultimately unanswerable, can be explored in therapy. Children's approaches to this can be highly variable. It may emerge in elaborate explanations of where the bug came from, involving aliens and spaceships, or in angry accusations at the doctors, reflecting a young child's confusion of cause and effect. One such child spontaneously drew an otherwise unexplained drawing entitled "Doctor jumping up and down on the man with the broken leg."

Guilt over imagined sins that might have caused this serious punishment, combined with the poor growth and emaciated body that hampers usual peer activities, can do serious damage to the child's self-esteem. One creative mother comforted her bright, artistic, but cachectic son with enough realistic, humorous, and loving support that he was able to create an "egghead" character. He used this character in therapy to reassure himself through stories and drawings that an unlikely looking man could still win friends with intelligence and kindness. Another young girl, too weak to attend school or other social activities, found self-esteem and satisfaction making paintings and other art projects for her parents and friends, even when too weak to hold a paintbrush without assistance.

A good working knowledge of the types of neuropsychologic deficits seen in children with AIDS allows the therapist to dispel attributions of laziness or oppositional behavior, improving self-perception as well as family interactions. With creativity and a good working relationship, the therapist and parents can help the child enjoy being alive, while fighting to make that life as long and healthy as it can be.

## Multiple Diagnoses in a Family

Seventy-nine percent of the reported cases of pediatric AIDS were acquired through vertical transmission, from mother to child (Gayle et al. 1990). Thus, for the vast majority of cases, children with HIV or AIDS are seen in a context where one or both parents are also infected. The medical and societal implications of this fact are staggering, as has been examined in several previous chapters. The psychotherapeutic issues are also many, and complex. There are very few disease processes that simultaneously affect both parent and child. Even therapists accustomed to working with other progressive, fatal illnesses may find the multiply infected family too tragic, and the issues too overwhelming. This is a powerful argument for a team approach (Stuber 1989). The family's treatment is simplified and coordinated by having one group medically manage both mother and child. The team should include two or more mental health professionals who can divide up responsibilities when appropriate (e.g., one working with the parents, the other seeing the child) or simply offer each other support and perspective. This permits the therapists some recovery time and distance when needed before plunging back into intense work with a dying family.

Parents often become very active and educated about their chronically ill child's care. Although most physicians find this helpful, some are uncomfortable with very assertive parents. (See Chapter 9, this volume, for further discussion of this issue.) Psychotherapists can help parents voice their concerns in a way that is most likely to get a result (persistent, but not attacking), while assisting the treatment team in managing their own guilt and defensiveness about not having the answers the parents want—an effective treatment or cure.

The degree of parental involvement required in all aspects of the infected child's physical care can also lead to intrusive, overprotective behavior from the parents, as well as dependency, hypochondriasis, and anxiety in the child. Such responses, although quite understandable, interfere with the child's ability to function at an optimal and developmentally appropriate level. They can also make treatment even more difficult, adding stress to clinic visits and confounding assessment of pain or medication side effects. This is particularly problematic when the child is the only member of the multiply infected family who is symptomatic. The child's symptoms and their treatment often become the focal point of the anxiety of an entire family. Mental health intervention can be extremely useful in refocusing some of this energy, allowing the family and the medical team to have a better working relationship (Krener 1987).

Treatment teams also become concerned when they notice that an infected mother is consistent and assertive about the treatment of her ill child, but appears to be ignoring her own health. The mental health specialist can point out that this is not particularly unusual behavior for mothers, who generally expect to put their child's welfare before their own. Psychologic and physical energy limitations may mean that only one illness can be attended to at a time. It may also be simply too overwhelming for the woman to acknowledge her own medical status while working to save the life of her child. Denial, even at the cost of the mother's own health care, may be more tolerable than the consistent awareness of her double vulnerability. This must be respected as an adaptive coping response, while the mental health specialist works with the family to help optimize the mental and physical well-being of all of its members (Stuber 1990).

Marital strain is common in families dealing with AIDS, as with other chronic illnesses. There are multiple reasons for this. Time, energy, and money that were previously available for adult activities are now taken up by health care. Parents are likely to differ in their style of coping, leading to disagreements and irritation. A typical example: one parent copes through information gathering, keeping voluminous notes and an ongoing list of questions for the physicians, whereas the other parent prefers a bit more denial and dependence on the medical team. Each finds the other's approach disturbing. The two parents are consequently unable to talk to each other at any length and cannot find support in one another. This scenario is common to many types of childhood illness. The problem is exacerbated in the case of pediatric AIDS for two reasons: 1) the parents often have no other supports with whom to discuss the illness, because it is not public knowledge, and 2) the child's illness is often blamed on one or the other of the parents, who is seen as having brought the virus into the family. The isolation and strain of the former situation have been discussed in earlier chapters. The latter problem, however, raises an aspect of pediatric AIDS that can be particularly pernicious: the question of blame.

Children with AIDS are commonly referred to as "innocent victims." It is easy to infer that whoever gave them this dread virus is the guilty perpetrator. Mothers, inclined to feel inadequate as parents simply for "allowing" their children to get sick, are especially prone to guilt if they are the vector by which the virus was passed on. Shifting the blame to the man who she believes infected her (either sexually or with shared drug "works") appears a reasonable alternative to the crushing guilt of being solely responsible for her child's death. The resulting accusations can lead to either an underlying tension or open confrontations as to who brought the virus into the family.

The blame can take on larger meaning as individuals try to answer the associated question of "Why me?" Repeated polls in the *Los Angeles Times* consistently found approximately one-fourth of the respondents agreeing that "AIDS is a punishment God has given homosexuals for the way they live" (28% on December 5, 1985; 24% on July 9, 1986; and 27% on July 24, 1987) (Herek and Glunt 1988). Attributing higher meaning to events in our lives is common to humankind, particularly when faced with catastrophic events. Psychotherapists can assist individuals and families as they search for meaning, trying to find an aspect that can allow growth, and not just suffering.

Although most therapists will at least attempt to take a neutral stance regarding blame within an infected family, it can be more difficult when the woman's serostatus is known before the birth of her child. If it is early enough in the pregnancy, the question of abortion is almost inevitably raised by medical or mental health professionals. The probability of transmission from mother to child, as discussed in Chapter 1, is less than 50%. Because these odds are far better than those for the mother's survival, many women feel the risk of having an infected child is tolerable in exchange for the chance to have a part of them survive (Selwyn et al. 1989).

Those familiar with the enormous suffering and expense of the brief lives of infected neonates often disagree. The resulting conflict has led some HIV-positive women to be secretive about their plans to conceive, sharing the news of their pregnancy only after it is too late to abort, resulting in inadequate health care for both mother and child (Selwyn et al. 1989). The best solution to this dilemma will be to find a way to prevent transmission of virus from mother to fetus. Research in this area is proceeding, but it is too early to know when or if it will be successful.

The uncertainty of a newborn's diagnosis (discussed in Chapter 1) further complicates a relationship already endangered by the chronic but progressive illness of the mother. The potential impact on bonding and early child rearing is enormous, but largely unexplored. A partial reason for the lack of good studies in this area is the confounding variable of foster care. Many infected mothers used drugs during pregnancy. Because this is considered child abuse in many states, it is not unusual for these newborns to be placed in protective custody, as wards of the court, shortly after birth. If the mother's situation is relatively stable, the child is returned after a few months. However, if the mother's medical status or neuropsychologic deterioration is sufficiently severe, or if for other reasons she is not able to care for the child, foster care placement continues. Mental health professionals can make significant interventions by working with the court or foster care system to help optimize the opportunity for good, stable nurturing relationships for these often difficult children.

Neonatal manifestations of HIV infection can, however, appear relatively rapidly, with children showing rapid deterioration within weeks to months. In some cases, the illness and resulting diagnosis will be the first indication that the mother might be infected. Thus, the family receives multiple diagnoses simultaneously. One such family, changing their self-concept from proud new parents and child to three dying individuals within a matter of days, became acutely suicidal. Urgent intervention was necessary to communicate some realistic hope and allow consideration of alternative options.

The wish to protect children from the grim realities of AIDS is a source of conflict for many families with multiple diagnoses. However, as discussed earlier, this may create as many problems as it solves. For example, a family with a symptomatic infected mother and a dying infant wished to hide the diagnosis from the (uninfected) school-age sibling and therefore avoided all discussion about the illness or treatment. However, when the older child was given a forum in which to talk about his situation, it was clear that he was extremely frightened and confused about what was happening in his family. It was necessary to assure him that he was not also going to get sick, and that, whatever happened to his mother, he would have a place to stay and someone to care for him. The same general principles apply that were discussed for the infected child: developmentally appropriate information, directed toward the areas of concern to the child, repeatedly stated by trusted adults.

Our distress as clinicians in dealing with these multiple tragedies can sometimes interfere with our ability to assess a situation. For example, a school-age child who had not been told that her mother's death had been due to AIDS began experiencing odd infectious diseases. No one expected the girl's HIV test to come back positive, so when it did the medical team was quite upset. Because it was felt that she was too old to be only now manifesting congenitally acquired AIDS, the psychiatric consultant was asked to find out from the child whether she had been sexually abused. Although the answer to this question was obviously important in establishing the etiology of the child's infection, some discussion clarified that this was probably not the most immediate issue for the child. The anguish of the team over having to simultaneously reveal to this child her own and her mother's diagnosis had overwhelmed their ability to think through a more gradual assessment, which would allow the child to process the information.

## Summary

Psychotherapeutic issues of pediatric AIDS range from assisting at-risk individuals to move beyond denial or counterphobic behavior, to working with the complex and emotionally draining realities of multiply infected families. Although many aspects of the actual interventions should be familiar to therapists experienced in work with adolescents or with seriously chronically ill children, there are additional elements that complicate and intensify the work. The stigma, isolation, secrecy, and ultimately fatal outcome that currently plague children with HIV infection will hopefully become only a tragic chapter in pediatric history as treatment and prevention efforts advance. However, for the present, psychotherapists who are able to take on the challenge of pediatric AIDS have a great deal to offer, both to their patients and to the community at large. Every bit of rationality and compassion that can be facilitated, whether with individuals, families, institutions, or the government, is a contribution toward a mentally healthy approach to pediatric AIDS.

Psychotherapists are not immune to irrational fears or biases and must themselves actively examine and combat the impulse to see HIV as a punishment or curse, and those who are infected as untouchable, evil, or pathetic (McKusick 1988). Even therapists experienced in work with AIDS patients catch themselves being casual about secretion precautions with patients who are not members of "high-risk groups" and meticulous with those we consider to be "at risk." It is difficult to always practice universal precautions. It is even more difficult to *think* in those terms. Both therapist and patient may feel uncomfortable when expected to assess all behavior in terms of risk for AIDS or other dangers. Unfortunately, this is what is necessary. It is only when we are able to understand and manage the resistance and prejudice in ourselves that we will be able to assist our patients to realistically assess the risk and act accordingly.

## References

Belfer ML, Krener PK, Miller FB: AIDS in children and adolescents. J Am Acad Child Adolesc Psychiatry 27:147–151, 1988

Bombeck E: I Want to Grow Hair, I Want to Grow Up, I Want to Go to Boise: Children Surviving Cancer. New York, Harper Collins, 1989

Gallo RC, Montagnier L: AIDS in 1988. Sci Am 259:41–48, 1988

Gayle JA, Selik RM, Chu SY: Surveillance for AIDS and HIV infection among black and Hispanic children and women of childbearing age, 1981–1989. MMWR 39 (SS-3):23–30, 1990

Herek GM, Glunt EK: An epidemic of stigma. Am Psychol 43:886–898, 1988

Katz ER, Ingle-Nelson MJ: School and the seriously ill child, in Pediatric Hospice Care: What Helps. Edited by Martin BB. Los Angeles, CA, Children's

Hospital, 1989, pp 145–167. Available from Belinda Martin, c/o Nursing Administration, #23, P.O. Box 54700, Los Angeles, CA 90054-0700

Kermani EJ: Handicapped children and the law: children afflicted with AIDS. J Am Acad Child Adolesc Psychiatry 27:152–154, 1988

Krener PG: Impact of the diagnosis of AIDS on hospital care of an infant. Clin Pediatr 26:30–34, 1987

McKusick L: The impact of AIDS on practitioner and client. Am Psychol 43:935–947, 1988

Selwyn PA, Schoenbaum EE, Davenny K, et al: Prospective study of human immunodeficiency virus infection and pregnancy outcomes in intravenous drug users. JAMA 261:1289–1294, 1989

Share L: Family communication in the crisis of a child's fatal illness: a literature review and analysis. Omega 3:3–10, 1972

Slavin LA, O'Malley JE, Koocher GP, et al: Communication of the cancer diagnosis to pediatric patients: impact on long-term adjustment. Am J Psychiatry 134:179–183, 1982

Sontag S: AIDS and Its Metaphors. New York, Vintage, 1989

Spinetta JJ: The dying child's awareness of death: a review. Psychol Bull 81:256–260, 1974

Stuber ML: Coordination of care for pediatric AIDS: the development of a maternal-child HIV task force. Dev Behav Pediatr 10:201–204, 1989

Stuber ML: Psychiatric consultation issues in pediatric HIV and AIDS. J Am Acad Child Adolesc Psychiatry 29:463–466, 1990

# Bibliography

## Books

*AIDS and Persons With Developmental Disabilities: The Legal Perspective.* American Bar Association, AIDS/DD Project, 1800 M Street, N.W., Washington, DC 20036; $18.00. 109-page report on legal issues of pediatric AIDS, including antidiscrimination statutes, HIV testing, informed consent, confidentiality, provider liability, isolation and involuntary civil commitment, and federal benefit and entitlement programs.

*AIDS: What Young Adults Should Know.* American Alliance for Health, Physical Education, Recreation and Dance, 1900 Association Drive, Reston, VA 22091. Education manual for instructors.

*Does AIDS Hurt?* M. Quackenbush, M.S., S. Villarrel, M.D. Network Publications, Santa Cruz, CA, 1988; $14.95. Comprehensive book about AIDS written for adults who care for young children. Includes discussions of age-appropriate answers to questions and AIDS education in the classroom.

*My Friend and AIDS.* S. Schilling and M. Mossberg. A Way With Words, P.O. Box 935, Parker, CO 80134; (303) 841-5497; $9.95. Written for children kindergarten through 3rd grade and their parents. Tells story of a friendship between Mark (an 8-year-old with hemophilia and HIV) and Josh. Includes photographs and facts about AIDS.

*My Name Is Jonathan (and I Have AIDS).* S. Schilling and J. Swain. Prickly Pair Publishing and Consulting Company, 9628 W. Oregon Place, Denver, CO 80226; (303) 986-3505. Paperback written for elementary school–age children about an elementary school boy with AIDS acquired through a neonatal transfusion. Thoughtful and helpful. Available in Spanish. Has a teacher's guide for use in classrooms.

*Someone at School Has AIDS: A Guide to Developing Policies for Students and School Staff Members Who Are Infected With HIV.* National Association of State Boards of Education (NASBE), Publications Department, 1012 Cameron Street, Alexandria, VA 22314; (703) 684-4000. Addresses infection control, confidentiality, and HIV-antibody testing.

*Teaching AIDS.* (Revised 1988). Marcia Quackenbush and Pamela Sargent. Network Publications, a Division of ETR Associates, P.O. Box 1830, Santa Cruz, CA 95061-1830 (ISBN 0-941816-41-9). An instructional manual.

*Workbook for the 5th National Pediatric AIDS Conference* and the follow-up to the 1987 Surgeon General's Workshop on Children With HIV Infection and Their Families. Available from Dr. John J. Hutchings, Office of Maternal and Child Health, Room 9-34, 5600 Fishers Lane, Rockville, MD 20857; (301) 443-2350.

## Newsletters

*Children With AIDS Newsletter.* Foundation for Children With AIDS, Inc., 77B Warren Street, Brighton, MA 02135; (617) 783-7300; $25 per year. Newsletter on research, clinical practices, and service delivery efforts.

*Disability Rights Education and Defense Funds News.* Contact DREDF Offices at 2112 Sixth Street, Berkeley, CA 94710; (415) 644-2555; or 1616 P Street, Suite 100, Washington, DC 20036; (202) 328-5185. Covers school and legal issues for people with disabilities, including those related to HIV.

## *Other*

American Academy of Child and Adolescent Psychiatry HIV Issues Committee. Contact Jacqueline Etemad, M.D., P.O. Box 37, Tiburon, CA 94920. Outlines recommendations for practicing child psychiatrists working with AIDS and HIV.

Information on clinical trials: Call 1-800-TRIALS-A to get written updates on currently available clinical trials. Very useful.

Pediatric AIDS Foundation, 2407 Wilshire Boulevard, Suite 613, Santa Monica, CA 90403; (213) 395-9051. Films, videos, educational materials, and other resources available for parents, children, and educators.

Spanish AIDS-related materials: Materials currently being identified, adapted, and translated by the Georgetown University Child Development Center AIDS Project, the National Institute of Drug Abuse, and the Pan American Health Organization (PAHO). Call PAHO at (915) 581-6645 or Diane Doherty at Georgetown at (202) 364-4164 for more information.